The Dilemma of Ritual Abuse

Cautions and Guides for Therapists

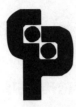

Judith H. Gold, M.D., F.R.C.P.C.
Elissa P. Benedek, M.D.
Series Editors

The Dilemma of Ritual Abuse

Cautions and Guides for Therapists

Edited by
George A. Fraser, M.D., F.R.C.P.C.

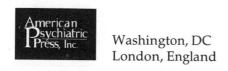

Washington, DC
London, England

Note: The authors have worked to ensure that all information in this book concerning drug dosages, schedules, and routes of administration is accurate as of the time of publication and consistent with standards set by the U.S. Food and Drug Administration and the general medical community. As medical research and practice advance, however, therapeutic standards may change. For this reason and because human and mechanical errors sometimes occur, we recommend that readers follow the advice of a physician who is directly involved in their care or the care of a member of their family.

Books published by the American Psychiatric Press, Inc., represent the views and opinions of the individual authors and do not necessarily represent the policies and opinions of the Press or the American Psychiatric Association.

Copyright © 1997 American Psychiatric Press, Inc.
ALL RIGHTS RESERVED
Manufactured in the United States of America on acid-free paper
First Edition   00   99   98   97   4   3   2   1

American Psychiatric Press, Inc.
1400 K Street, N.W., Washington, DC 20005

Library of Congress Cataloging-in-Publication Data
The dilemma of ritual abuse : cautions and guides for therapists /
    edited by George A. Fraser. — 1st ed.
        p.   cm. — (Clinical practice ; no. 41)
    Includes bibliographical references and index.
    ISBN 0-88048-478-0 (alk. paper)
    1. Ritual abuse victims—Rehabilitation.   I. Fraser, George A.,
    1941–   .   II. Series.
    [DNLM: 1. Multiple-Personality Disorder—therapy.   2. Child Abuse—
    psychology.   3. Occultism.   4. Ceremonial.   W1 CL767J no.41 1997 /
    WM 173.6 D576 1997]
    RC569.5.R59D55   1997
    616.85′82—DC20
    DNLM/DLC
    for Library of Congress   96-30140
                                                                               CIP

British Library Cataloguing in Publication Data
A CIP record is available from the British Library.

Contents

I

Clinical Experience

II

Special Techniques and Issues

Contributors

Joseph Barber, Ph.D.
Associate Clinical Professor, Departments of Anesthesiology and
Rehabilitation Medicine, School of Medicine, University of
Washington, Seattle

Suzette Boon, Ph.D.
Clinical Psychologist and Psychotherapist, Dissociation Team, Regional
Institute of Ambulatory Mental Health Care South/New West,
Amsterdam, The Netherlands

John M. W. Bradford, M.D., F.R.C.P.C.
Professor of Psychiatry, University of Ottawa Medical School; Director,
Forensic Program, and Director, Sexual Behaviours Clinic, Royal
Ottawa Hospital, Ontario

Bennett G. Braun, M.D.
Director, Section of Psychiatric Trauma, Rush-Presbyterian-St. Luke's
Medical Center, Chicago, Illinois; Medical Director, Dissociative
Disorders Program, Rush North Shore Medical Center, Skokie, Illinois

Philip M. Coons, M.D.
Professor of Psychiatry, Indiana University School of Medicine,
Indianapolis, Indiana

George A. Fraser, M.D., F.R.C.P.C.
Assistant Professor of Psychiatry, University of Ottawa Medical School;
Director, Anxiety and Phobic Disorders Clinic, Royal Ottawa Hospital,
Ottawa, Ontario

Olga Heijtmajer Jansen, M.D.
Private practice in psychiatry, Amsterdam, The Netherlands

Richard P. Kluft, M.D.
Director, Dissociative Disorders Program, Institute of Pennsylvania
Hospital; Clinical Professor of Psychiatry, Temple University School of
Medicine, Philadelphia, Pennsylvania; Lecturer in Psychiatry, Harvard
Medical School, Cambridge, Massachusetts

Stephen S. Marmer, M.D., Ph.D.
Private practice in psychiatry and psychoanalysis; Clinical Faculty,
Department of Psychiatry, University of California at Los Angeles
School of Medicine, Los Angeles, California

Robert J. Simandl
International Police Consultant and Police Officer, Chicago Police
Department, Chicago, Illinois

Onno van der Hart, Ph.D.
Chief, Trauma and Dissociation Team, Regional Institute of
Ambulatory Mental Health Care South/New West, Amsterdam;
Professor, Department of Clinical and Health Psychology, Utrecht
University, Utrecht, The Netherlands

Linda J. Young, R.N.C., M.A.
Head Nurse, Ft. Lyon Veterans Administration Hospital, Ft. Lyon,
Colorado; Former Clinical Director, National Treatment Center for
Dissociative Disorders, Del Amo Hospital, Torrance, California

Walter C. Young, M.D., F.A.P.A.
Assistant Chief of Staff, Psychiatry, Ft. Lyon Veterans Administration
Hospital, Ft. Lyon, Colorado; Former Medical Director, National
Treatment Center for Dissociative Disorders, Del Amo Hospital,
Torrance, California

Introduction

to the Clinical Practice Series

Over the years of its existence the series of monographs entitled *Clinical Insights* gradually became focused on providing current, factual, and theoretical material of interest to the clinician working outside of a hospital setting. To reflect this orientation, the name of the Series has been changed to *Clinical Practice*.

The Clinical Practice Series will provide books that give the mental health clinician a practical, clinical approach to a variety of psychiatric problems. These books will provide up-to-date literature reviews and emphasize the most recent treatment methods. Thus, the publications in the Series will interest clinicians working both in psychiatry and in the other mental health professions.

Each year a number of books will be published dealing with all aspects of clinical practice. In addition, from time to time when appropriate, the publications may be revised and updated. Thus, the Series will provide quick access to relevant and important areas of psychiatric practice. Some books in the Series will be authored by a person considered to be an expert in that particular area; others will be edited by such an expert, who will also draw together other knowledgeable authors to produce a comprehensive overview of that topic.

Some of the books in the Clinical Practice Series will have their foundation in presentations at an annual meeting of the American Psychiatric Association. All will contain the most recently available information on the subjects discussed. Theoretical and scientific data will be applied to clinical situations, and case illustrations will be utilized in order to make the material even more relevant for the practitioner. Thus, the Clinical Practice Series should provide educational reading in a compact format especially designed for the mental health clinician–psychiatrist.

Judith H. Gold, M.D., F.R.C.P.C.
Series Editor

Introduction

George A. Fraser, M.D., F.R.C.P.C.

*T*his book is for the therapist and others interested in the ritual abuse (RA) phenomenon. It is not an attempt to prove or disprove the reality of ritualized abuse; rather, it is hoped to be a guide to therapists. Clinical experience indicates that not all reports of RA are accurate. History and the legal profession will clarify whether some reports may be partially or wholly accurate. In the meantime, despite the ongoing controversy, clinicians continue to have patients seeking help for recollections they believe point to ritualized abuses earlier in their lives. The reader will find in this book a group of well-qualified and experienced authors who offer advice on approaches that should be considered when a therapist faces a patient presenting with a history containing elements pertaining to abuses in satanic and/or sadistic ritualized settings.

Were this book written in the mid-1980s, a marked polarity of opinions by the authors would have been likely. While there do remain, in the late 1990s, protagonists who debate with passion for one or the other side of the RA veracity issue, I was nonetheless struck by the more balanced viewpoints as the chapters independently arrived from these authors. Such balanced thinking seems to reflect the current thinking of those seriously studying the dilemma of RA.

There is, however, little formal research into the RA phenomenon. Many of the authors of this book are very active in the evaluation and therapy of patients reporting RAs. These chapters are the personal opinions of these authors. It is unavoidable when dealing with a limited topic that there will be some overlap among chapters; nonetheless, each chapter offers its own important message to guide the therapist evaluating RA reports.

The term *ritual abuse* was probably first used in the book *Michelle Remembers* (Smith and Pazder 1980), in which the recovered memories of a patient are recounted. Other more recent terms used for this phenomenon are *sadistic abuse* (Goodwin 1993), *satanic ritual abuse* (Van Benschoten 1990), and *sadistic ritual abuse*. The acronym SRA is used for both these latter two terms, whereas RA may refer to either ritual abuse, ritualistic abuse (Kluft 1989), or ritualized abuse. Throughout the book, one or another of these terms is used depending on the author. No one of these terms seems acceptable to everyone. Because *ritual abuse* seems most commonly used, this term was finally chosen to be used in the title of the book. For the most part, these terms could be looked upon as essentially interchangeable in this collection. As psychiatry attempts to focus on the group abuse issues rather than the satanic rituals, newer terms are being used, including *organized abuse* and *organized sadistic abuse*. No matter which term is used, sadism and exploitation are reportedly key elements to this abuse phenomenon.

RA can have many interpretations depending on the culture and context in which it is used (Greaves 1992). Not all RA is satanic, nor are groups practicing satanism as a religion necessarily involved in RA. The term in this book, in most but not all cases, refers to abuses said to be done in satanic ceremonies. Alleged activities in these reports of RA include the following phenomena:

- Perverted physical, psychological, and sexual abuse of children and adults is reported in groups frequently claiming or pretending to worship Satan.
- Mind coercion techniques, including terror and isolation, are reportedly used to obtain compliance, discourage defection, and ensure future obedience, allegiance, and secrecy.
- Enforced membership lasts for many years, lasting ideally for life.
- Members may believe themselves wedded or committed to Satan and unable to escape his ever-watchful eye.
- There is obedience to a hierarchy of leadership. Leaders are often called priests or priestesses.
- Ceremonies are said to include the ingestion of blood and urine obtained from humans or animals.

- Human sacrifices allegedly occur, and human body parts may be disposed of in ritualized cannibalistic ceremonies.
- Inbreeding and the subsequent desecration of the fetus or newborn are reported. In other cases, some infants are supposedly groomed as future leaders or recruiters.
- Members may come from all strata of society. Multigenerational familial participation is said to be common.
- Sexual orgies, including pedophilia, promiscuity, and bestiality, reportedly take place. Frequently these acts are done under the influence of mind-altering chemicals. These acts may be filmed for future sale in the pornographic market.
- Ceremonies supposedly occur on major Christian feast days or on days relating to natural planetary phases such as the summer solstice or the cycles of the moon.

Reports of patients recalling RA dramatically increased around the mid-1980s. These reports mostly came from patients who were already in therapy for repressed or dissociated memories of childhood abuse who had been diagnosed as having multiple personality disorder (MPD), one of the dissociative disorders in DSM-III-R (American Psychiatric Association 1987). In DSM-IV (American Psychiatric Association 1994), MPD is renamed dissociative identity disorder (DID).

As these dramatic stories of abuse began to surface, some therapists believed RA to be the ultimate form of sexual and physical abuse. However, others became quite skeptical and began to question the reality of these so-called recollections (Ganaway 1989). Books covering many of the issues of RA include *The Satanism Scare* (Richardson et al. 1991), *Out of Darkness: Exploring Satanism and Ritual Abuse* (Sakheim and Devine 1992), and *Satanic Ritual Abuse: Principles of Treatment* (Ross 1995). There are various good sources, many of which are included in the reference lists of the authors in this book. I also recommend the special issues of *International Journal of Clinical and Experimental Hypnosis* on "Hypnosis and Delayed Recall" (Frankel and Perry 1994) and *Journal of Psychohistory* on "Backlash Against Psychotherapy" (Winter 1995), as well as *Clinical Hypnosis and Memory: Guidelines for Clinicians and for Forensic Hypnosis* (American Society of Clinical Hypnosis 1995).

Police agencies became involved when numerous reports of burials of sacrificed children and dismembered bodies arose. The U.S. Federal Bureau of Investigation and other agencies found no such evidence (Lanning 1992). The legal system also was involved later when patients having recollections of parental collusion in the satanic RAs began taking their parents to court, based on memories elicited during therapy. Alarm grew among those who claimed they were being falsely accused.

In 1992, a group of parents formed the False Memory Syndrome Foundation (FMSF) to assist those stating they were falsely accused. The FMSF believes, among other things, that misguided therapists led patients into the misbelief that they had been ritually abused and states such therapists should be accountable to the courts. The media, which had sensationalized the initial reports of RA, now embraced this counterclaim. Therapists found themselves caught in a backlash of public opinion. They were now portrayed as the cause of the phenomenon (Quirk and DePrince 1995).

Those not involved in the problem, or reviewing the topic of RA at a later time, may comment on the naïveté of those grappling with this issue. However, it is very different to actually face a new and urgent phenomenon and deal with it, but not fully understand it, while managing distressed and confused patients and their families.

On the positive side, the RA issue has caused us to take a closer look at issues of trauma, hypnosis, memory, and memory recall. The FMSF has cited work of scientists who point out that memory is subject to distortion (Loftus 1993). Although the possibility of hypnotically refreshed recall of memories being false was noted (American Medical Association 1985), it unfortunately was forgotten or ignored by some therapists. For various reasons, they were too keen to embrace these recollections of repressed or dissociated memories as totally reliable.

The influence a therapist has on a patient should not be forgotten. Expectation and subtle (even subliminal) cues by the therapist may create or guide the response given by the patient. This influence has long been well known to the field of hypnosis. One should be aware of the potential difficulties in using hypnosis and related techniques, such as guided imagery and Sodium Amytal interviews, in memory recall. Not only can these techniques result in contaminated memories, but they could render the patient ineligible for a subsequent court case (Scheflin 1993; Scheflin and Shapiro 1989). Therapists are now being advised to consider having a consent form signed by patients advising them of the difficulties in refreshed memory techniques and warning them of the possibility that they may be unable to engage in a future related court case if hypnosis is used. Consent forms might protect the therapist from a future lawsuit (Scheflin 1993) by the patient. In 1993, the American Psychiatric Association issued a "Statement on Memories of Sexual Abuse." (See the Appendix for the complete text of this statement.)

The fields of trauma and posttraumatic stress disorder have much to offer in comprehending the phenomenon of RA. Those supporting the possibility of the accuracy of memory recall have cited a recent publication of van der Kolk (1994) concerning posttraumatic stress disorder in which he noted that certain forms of somatosensory memory recorded during trauma (implicit memory) may bypass hippocampal processing and be stored in a different manner than normal (explicit) memory. He states that initial recall of these traumatic implicit memories may be quite accurate (van der Kolk 1994). More explorations into this area are needed before final conclusions are drawn.

Though recalled memories may be false, studies by researchers (e.g., Kluft 1995; Williams 1992) indicate that repression or dissociation of traumatic events does happen, and recall years later can indeed be accurate. However, we as therapists do not necessarily know how to distinguish between true and false memories. This difficulty in discerning an absolute truth must be kept in mind during therapy and in advising patients who might consider litigation based solely on recovered memories.

Certainly one of the arguments against RA in satanic settings has been the lack of criminal convictions. Yet in 1995, a Reuters News Agency article reported an actual conviction that year in Europe. The article, originating in Athens, Greece, begins as follows:

> The leaders of a satanic cult which conducted human sacrifices on the outskirts of Athens were sentenced to life in prison yesterday for the rape and murder of two women in a grisly case that mesmerized Greece. ("Greece Jails 3 for Life" 1995, p. A10)

The sentence of the 20-year-old "high priestess" was reduced to 18 years and 4 months because of "her young age at the time of the crimes." It was reported that the three main defendants "confessed after their arrest in December 1993 that they led a 20-member satanic cult, which conducted animal and human sacrifices, for three years" (p. A10). The investigator who solved the case in 1994 doubted that the activities were a true religious practice and from his investigation concluded that "Satanism was an excuse to get sick sex and money" (p. A10).

Even as this book goes to press, the dilemma of ritual abuse continues to be current and perplexing. In the summer of 1996, the world awoke to the news of the gruesome pedophilic murder of a number of children in Belgium. In January 1997, Dr. Onno van der Hart, a contributor to this book, sent to me a copy of *The Sunday Times* (London), which contained an article headlined "Satanic Links to Belgian Murder Trial." The article begins as follows:

> Satanic sects involved in bizarre human sacrifices are being linked by Belgian police with this summer's string of grisly pedophile murders in which at least four children died.
>
> Five witnesses came forward last week and described how black masses were held, at which children were killed in front of audiences said to have included prominent members of Belgian society. One investigator said it was "like going back to the Middle Ages." (Conrad 1996, p. 14)

Although a newspaper article is hardly a source of unquestionable accuracy, it nonetheless points out that the problem of ritual abuse is far from over, and therapists need to become educated about this phenomenon when called upon for help, advice, and cautions.

This book was written at the time DSM-IV changed the term *multiple personality disorder* to *dissociative identity disorder*. Because the former term is still used in many parts of the world, I retained the terms used by the authors.

There is a caution for readers: Some may find certain chapters and drawings upsetting because of their subject matter. If you as a reader are concerned that this book may be disturbing, please discuss this concern with a colleague or therapist before reading it.

I deeply thank the contributing authors for having the courage to present their ideas on this very difficult topic. I hope that this book contributes to a better understanding and respect among those holding opposing viewpoints on RA by providing a balanced guide for therapists struggling to understand the dilemma of RA. Putnam (1991) voiced a wish for disciplines to work in tandem to help clarify this conundrum without causing further harm either to therapists or to patients. I sincerely hope that therapists, patients, and their families will benefit from the work of the authors of this book.

I also thank the following co-workers for their help in preparing the text: Lynn Bourdon, Susan Fazzino, Jane W. Fraser, Dayle Raine, and Suzanne M. Fraser. Finally, special thanks to my family who allowed me to spend many of my spare hours working on this project: Freda, Jane-Diane, Suzanne, Sean, Hilda, Calum, and Rowan.

References

American Medical Association Council on Scientific Affairs: Council report: scientific status of refreshing recollection by the use of hypnosis. JAMA 253:1918–1923, 1985

American Psychiatric Association: Diagnostic and Statistical Manual of Mental Disorders, 3rd Edition, Revised. Washington, DC, American Psychiatric Association, 1987

American Psychiatric Association: Diagnostic and Statistical Manual of Mental Disorders, 4th Edition. Washington, DC, American Psychiatric Association, 1994

American Society of Clinical Hypnosis Committee on Hypnosis and Memory: Clinical Hypnosis and Memory: Guidelines for Clinicians and for Forensic Hypnosis. Des Plaines, IL, American Society of Clinical Hypnosis, 1995

Backlash Against Psychotherapy. Journal of Psychohistory, Vol 22, No 3 (special issue), 1995

Conrad P: Satanic links to Belgian murder trial. The Sunday Times, December 29, 1996, p 14

Frankel FH, Perry CW (eds): Hypnosis and Delayed Recall, I. Int J Clin Exp Hypn, Vol 42, No 4 (special issue), 1994

Ganaway GK: Historical truth versus narrative truth: clarifying the role of exogenous trauma in the etiology of multiple personality disorder and its variants. Dissociation 2:205–220, 1989

Goodwin JM: Human vectors of trauma: illustrations from the Marquis de Sade, in Rediscovering Childhood Trauma: Historical Casebook and Clinical Applications. Edited by Goodwin JM. Washington, DC, American Psychiatric Press, 1993, pp 95–111

Greece jails 3 for life in satanic slayings. Toronto Star, July 1, 1995, p A10

Greaves GB: Alternative hypotheses regarding claims of satanic cult activity: a critical analysis, in Out of Darkness: Exploring Satanism and Ritual Abuse. Edited by Sakheim DK, Devine SE. New York, Lexington Books, 1992, pp 45–72

Kluft RP: Editorial: reflection on allegations of ritual abuse. Dissociation 2:191–193, 1989

Kluft RP: The confirmation and disconfirmation of memories of abuse in dissociative identity patients: a naturalistic clinical study. Dissociation 4:253–258, 1995

Lanning K: Investigators Guide to Allegations of "Ritual" Child Abuse. Washington, DC, U.S. Federal Bureau of Investigation, 1992

Loftus EF: The reality of repressed memories. Am Psychol 48:518–537, 1993

Putnam FW: The satanic ritual abuse controversy. Child Abuse Negl 15:175–179, 1991

Quirk SA, DePrince AP: Backlash legislation targeting psychotherapists. Journal of Psychohistory 22:258–264, 1995

Richardson JT, Best J, Bromley DG (eds): The Satanism Scare. New York, Aldine de Gruyter, 1991

Ross CA: Satanic Ritual Abuse: Principles of Treatment. Toronto, Ontario, University of Toronto Press, 1995

Sakheim DK, Devine SE (eds): Out of Darkness: Exploring Satanism and Ritual Abuse. New York, Lexington Books, 1992

Scheflin AW: Avoiding malpractice liability. American Society of Clinical Hypnosis Newsletter, August 1993, p 6

Scheflin AW, Shapiro JL: Trance on Trial. New York, Guilford, 1989

Smith M, Pazder L: Michelle Remembers. New York, Pocket Books, 1980

Van Benschoten SC: Multiple personality disorder and satanic ritual abuse: the issue of credibility. Dissociation 3:22–30, 1990

van der Kolk BA: The body keeps the score: memory and evolving psychobiology of post-traumatic stress. Harvard Review of Psychiatry 1:253–265, 1994

Williams LM: Adult memories of childhood abuse: preliminary findings from a longitudinal study. The American Professional Society on the Abuse of Children Advisor, Summer 1992, pp 19–21

Section I

Clinical Experience

CHAPTER 1

A Credulous Skeptic's Approach to Cults and Multiple Personality Disorder

Stephen S. Marmer, M.D., Ph.D.

*L*istening to an archival recording of Edward R. Murrow's first broadcast from Buchenwald, I was struck by the power of his words and the intensity of his voice. I cannot recall his precise words, but he said in effect, "I know that few of you are going to believe this report, for what I am about to tell you defies common sense and goes beyond human experience; yet it is true, for I have seen it with my own eyes." He then went on to describe in vivid but sober phrases the evil horrors of the Holocaust's extermination camps. There are still those today who prefer not to believe what happened there, and I wonder what the world will be like when the last survivor and the last liberator pass from our midst.

Murrow's report rings in my ears whenever I think about the current controversy over satanic ritual abuse (SRA). After all, many of us treating patients with multiple personality disorder (MPD) have run into colleagues who did not believe that MPD existed. Just a few decades ago, prevailing learned opinion held that child abuse was a rare phenomenon—perhaps one in a million. I sat in a meeting at the American Psychiatric Association in 1972 when first films of acupuncture were shown to professional medical organizations. Most psychiatrists in the room did not believe what was shown on the films, and those who did believed that the phenomena were due to hypnosis or suggestion rather than to acupuncture itself. We know that sometimes things can happen that are very difficult to believe.

Many problems confront the investigator who wishes to address satanic ritual cult abuse and MPD. First, there is no Edward R. Murrow doing the reporting. He had an impeccable record of fairness and objectivity in his reporting and in his delivery of the news. He also had concrete and objective evidence to show the world. Both of these are lacking in the investigation of satanic ritual cult abuse; we have neither the calm fair reporter nor the concrete evidence for experts and the public to examine. Second, it is troubling that reports of satanic abuse began in the mid-1980s. Having seen my first patient with MPD in 1971, I did not hear a patient of mine with MPD report anything remotely resembling satanic abuse until 1987. Each of my patients who has reported satanic or cult abuse has previously heard stories of such matters from other patients before reporting it to me. None had retrieved independent memories of such abuse. Third, although reports of abduction and sexual abuse at the hands of alien extraterrestrials has not been an issue with any of my MPD patients, I have heard and seen such reports from cases I have consulted on or observed. These reports lead me to believe that not every report from a patient who has MPD or a history of childhood abuse is necessarily to be accepted at face value.

This phenomenon raises many questions of its own. We are used to believing the statements of our patients, and we are often in the position of supporting their quest to discover the truth about their past with an attitude of presuming the veracity of their memories and reports. We do this for the perfectly good reason that an atmosphere of acceptance fosters the therapeutic alliance and provides the empathic environment necessary for progress. Many therapists veer much more toward accepting the reports of their MPD patients than those of their non-MPD patients. A psychiatrist I know accepts at face value the reports of the childhood experiences of his MPD patients, while taking the position that the perspectives of his patients with schizophrenia, bipolar disorder, and borderline personality disorder are likely to be distorted or at least "spun" by the patients for psychodynamic reasons. The necessary corrective for the undue doubt that MPD patients face from their families, and that treaters of MPD face from doubting colleagues, can easily turn into unquestioning acceptance.

We know very well that human beings can distort their perceptions and their memories. Human beings are distinct from other creatures in the skill and extent to which they establish symbolic representation of their experience. Therapists skilled in the interpretation of symbols may tend to take MPD patients' reports as concrete and accurate recordings of events rather than as symbolic representations. This is the fourth problem confronting those investigating satanic ritual cult abuse and MPD. Although sometimes patients can have an astounding recall for their past, at other times their access to past memories and affects is mediated by symbolization, condensation, and displacement—the very ingredients producing dreams (Freud 1900/1953). Patients with dissociative disorders have the paradox of too much memory and not enough memory. They lose time and forget where they are going or who they are, but they have islands of intense flashback experiences in which they are trapped in memory. One dissociative patient of mine demonstrated this paradox when she could not remember her checkbook and was no longer able to memorize music (she was a professional musician), but she was able to recall the eight-digit serial number of a gun someone had used to threaten her 4 years earlier. She had glanced at the gun for no longer than 2 or 3 seconds, yet she was able to remember the serial number 4 years later during a flashback that took place on awakening from a dream. The Bureau of Alcohol, Tobacco, and Firearms in Washington, D.C., was able to confirm the correctness of that memory.

Yet when the famous Dr. Schreber remembered being called by God, with rays from the heavens, to change his sex and be impregnated by those rays so that he could populate the earth with a new race of people, we understood that he was speaking in metaphor and symbol and did not start an organization for those suffering from "God's Ray Abuse." The original analysis of Schreber's diary emphasized the psychodynamic relationship between Schreber and his father (Freud 1911/1958). Subsequent writers have researched the child-rearing practices in the Schreber family and concluded that the young Schreber had been a survivor of what we would now call childhood sexual and physical abuse (Niederland

1974). The relevance to this discussion is that Schreber symbolized the abuse from his father using the metaphor of rays from God (see also Spence 1982 and Schafer 1983; for another view, see Masson 1984). This metaphor for abuse is what I have found among those MPD patients in my practice who have remembered what they have called satanic ritual cult abuse.

Case Examples

Although I do not exclude the possibility that further evidence could confirm reports of a worldwide satanic conspiracy, as well as reports of alien extraterrestrial abductions for sexual abuse purposes, evidence from my own practice supports the view that, like Schreber, these patients are using satanic ritual cult abuse as a metaphor to defend against a more pressing danger. As these dangers are identified and worked through, my patients thus far have come to see their story of "satanic" activities as a way of deflecting something else. I present vignettes from five cases: one in which reports of satanic cults served to distance the patient from the reality of what her father and mother did; one in which the patient felt she had to have a compelling story of abuse to be taken seriously; two in which the recounting of satanic abuse helped the patients discover some real, but not satanic, group abuse activities; and one whose underlying character structure was hyperbolic and dramatic in all areas and across all personalities, leading to the exaggeration and dramatization of what was a real abuse history elaborated into a satanic story. In all of these cases I was prepared to be convinced of the veracity of the satanic stories, but in each instance the patient came to see her story in a different light, while gaining even greater clarity for the other abuse events in her life.

Case 1

Randi was 30 years old when she came to see me. She had been treated by a therapist in a different state who had become excessively fascinated by MPD and by the patient's memories, and in the course of her prior treatment, this overeager pouring forth of her story retraumatized her, requiring hospitalization. In a manic state during that hospitalization, Randi for the first time added details of satanic abuse to her story. When I saw her, she was depressed over the effects of the prior hospitalization, depressed over leaving (or more properly being dismissed) by her over-whelmed former therapist, and depressed over having to leave her former location to accommodate her husband's career.

At first she was dismayed by the slower pace of our work com-pared to the rapid pace of work with her former therapist. Her child alters sorely missed her prior therapist, but a good working alliance developed fairly soon. The main highlights of her history involved growing up in the early 1960s in a small suburb of a medium-sized city in a large state. Her father was a respected fire captain who provided for his family but was also an alcoholic who molested Randi starting when she was between ages 2 and 3. Randi attempted to alert her mother, who was unresponsive and perhaps intermittently psychotic. When Randi's younger sister turned age 3, Randi was forced by her father to bring the sister into the sexual activities. Randi did this in the belief that if the two children in the same family were being abused, surely someone would notice. She also needed company and someone to talk to about her experiences so that she wouldn't feel so alone. Her MPD became a problem that brought her into treatment when her own child reached age 3 and Randi felt that she might harm the child.

During therapy, whenever we focused on Randi's love for her father, her profoundly mixed feelings about being abused by the relatively more nurturing parent, about the loss of a protective mother, or about the guilt she felt for having brought her younger sister into the abuse system, she had intrusive thoughts of satanic ritual cult abuse. Sometimes her intrusive thoughts would take the form of two or three of her personalities interrupting the flow of our sessions with urgent memories or stories of their own. Sometimes personalities with no specific thoughts of satanic mat-ters would be flooded with body memories or auditory messages that she interpreted as satanic. She felt that the talk of her love for her father or the absence of her mother was triggering the body memories and that she was being punished by Satan for being disrespectful of her father's priestly position. She began to have less conviction about what happened in her nuclear family and more thoughts about rituals taking place in the nearby woods. She even wondered if she had been designated to become a priestess or a breeder, only to be pushed aside when her younger sister was perceived as a more gifted initiate. Instead of feeling guilty about bringing her sister to her father's room, she began to feel jealous of the extra attention her sister was getting from the cult. The cult practices turned out to be identical to those described by her roommate at the hospital.

As time went by, the pattern of satanic thoughts whenever we discussed her nuclear family became more and more consistent. One day a helper alter left a message on my answering machine telling me that none of the satanic rituals had happened and that Randi was using them as a distraction to keep away from feelings about her father and a growing compulsion to injure her own child. I had suspected this for some time but did not announce the telephone message to other alters. However, I took this telephone message as a sign that I could begin openly interpreting the satanic thoughts as a resistance. At first this resulted in worsening of Randi's symptoms. She had more body memories, severe headaches, trouble with her vision, and confusional states. At the time, I wondered whether this change in her symptoms represented worsening because I was moving away from important (satanic) material that had to be explored or whether it represented progress because we were moving away from distracting resistance (satanic) and toward truer material. My question was answered gradually as the nature of the affect over her father, mother, sister, and child became more and more poignant and intense. As I continued to focus my interpretations on exploring Randi's feelings about her relationship with her family, I did not express doubt about the satanic material; rather, as the alters began to feel the rage, sadness, despair, abandonment, competition, guilt, and dread, as well as the love and pleasure, of those primary relationships, the satanic material receded. Randi began to wonder whether it had really happened or whether she had made it up, with a growing conviction toward the latter.

Case 2

Patricia is an example of the pseudofalse positive that Kluft (1991) describes. At our first meeting, she brought a bagful of toys and props, which she said each of her alters needed to feel comfortable. She made a big fuss over switching alters, throwing her head back, stiffening her body, then coming to as the new alter. Each alter then went searching through her bag for the appropriate prop or toy. Some assumed caricatured accents; others had special glasses and complained that they were blind if they used another alter's glasses. I saw Patricia for six sessions as part of an extended evaluation consultation.

During each session, her behavior and her story escalated. The satanic material did not come up until the fourth session. When she saw that I was interested, she accommodated my interest with more detail in session five. In the sixth session, I expressed the opinion that she did indeed have MPD and that the overly flamboyant nature of her presentation contributed more than anything to my initial doubt that she had MPD.

I did not treat Patricia, and she remained in treatment with the next therapist for only 1½ years, until she was lost to my follow-up. However, the next therapist reported that as the work progressed, the flamboyant nature of the alters subsided and the satanic material disappeared altogether. Both appeared to be part of Patricia's effort to get help and thus were part of the false-positive syndrome. She had believed that unless her story was convincing, she would be dismissed or misdiagnosed, as had been the case on previous attempts to get treatment.

Case 3

Doris also came for a consultation. She was having intrusive thoughts and painful body memories. She was unusual in that she more closely resembled the MPD patients of an earlier era, with only four alters. She was a successful attorney in another part of California whose treating therapist requested a series of consultations with me during her treatment.

While exploring extremely painful and stimulating genitourinary body memories, Doris became convinced that she had been impregnated at age 12. Over the months, a story of SRA developed. She had visions of men in black robes holding upside-down crosses, sacrificing animals, and making children drink blood. She had the sense of hearing a child cry as it was sacrificed. She thought that she had been pregnant and had delivered a child. She had a strong sense of other neighborhood girls standing in a row with her at cult events, each made to drink various potions that drugged them. She was convinced that most of the girls in her school were involved in this cult and that the parents had an ongoing association with the cult. This conviction was all the more remarkable because Doris came from an ethnically Jewish, although completely assimilated and nonreligious, background and lived in the heart of a major urban area.

During her treatment, Doris contacted some of her childhood friends. Most of them rejected her and her story, but two were interested because they had vague memories of a child's death and of some kind of group activities. They were able to discover together that there had indeed been a group of radical bohemian parents who had libertine ideas about self-expression, sex, and pornography. The parents did meet for group sex, and sometimes the sexual experiences included teenage and preteen girls. There was also considerable experimentation with drugs among the parents, with alcohol and drugs sometimes being given to the children. There was no memory on the part of the other friends of anything satanic, and Doris concluded that her satanic material was an available template by which she could express part of the truth: there were group activities that she witnessed and may have participated in as a child. The death of the youngster may have occurred when the parents were in a drugged state. However, Doris's childhood experience does not appear to have been a part of a satanic ritual cult abuse conspiracy.

Case 4

Faith had dreams of a stone altar surrounded by gray crosses and black-robed men engaging in responsive chanting. This intrusive image was shared by several of her personalities, and it came out spontaneously in her drawing. She also dreamed and wrote of a cavern or room, which could be entered only by going down a long staircase, where she had been abused sexually and threatened physically by a group of men.

As treatment progressed, Faith realized that her mother and stepfather had both been severe alcoholics. Her stepfather had many drunken parties in the basement of their home. Finally, her mother and stepfather joined Alcoholics Anonymous (AA). After many relapses, they finally attained stable sobriety. Eventually, they became AA enthusiasts, earning the label of "guardian angels" of their meetings. However, the abuse of Faith continued, especially by the stepfather and his friends. She was threatened with severe bodily harm if she told anyone. Efforts to tell teachers through indirect methods, such as in stories she would write in her English classes, failed. When she joined AA as an adult, she quickly became involved sexually with AA men in the worst stages of incomplete recovery, and she found herself in many abusive situations.

Faith believed in AA and its effectiveness in keeping her and millions of others sober. So when memories of her mother and stepfather abusing her started to emerge, she placed them in a satanic context rather than an AA context to preserve the good relationship she had with AA. Only as she moved forward in her therapy did she feel enough inner unity and a strong enough hold on her sobriety to remove the disguise of SRA and see that there was indeed group abuse, but it was more personal and familial rather than satanic.

To be sure there is no misunderstanding, Faith's experience with certain abusive members of her parents' AA circle is not to be taken as a generalization about AA. Quite the contrary, Faith's more than 12 years of sobriety in AA has been lifesaving.

Case 5

According to Bibi, she has the most complex case of MPD there has ever been. She had worn out 10 psychiatrists, none of whom was as smart as she was, none of whom was capable of mastering the intricacies of her case. At the moment, she regards me as the one therapist on earth who is good enough to help her, although she takes pains to assure me that she is just as smart as I am, if not smarter. She regards it as a badge of her honor to be with "the best doctor on earth."

Members of her family who own stock in public companies are not mere stockholders; they "own" IBM, General Motors, and Citibank. All of her successful relatives operate the number one company of its type in the world. She was the best athlete in her school, her escapades were the most dangerous ever seen, her substance use the worst Dr. so-and-so had ever seen, her eating disorder the most amazing case such-and-such hospital had ever admitted. When a suicidal alter appears in a session, she is the most dangerously suicidal person I have ever seen. When an angry alter appears, she never has mere anger; she always has blinding rage. The flirtatious alter can get any man to do anything she wants. Her boyfriends are always the most handsome men ever, and several movie stars are on her list. Careless or risk-taking alters never get into ordinary car accidents; they always get into nearly fatal ones. When she suffers body memories, they last nonstop for 24 hours, with a combination of stimulation that is poised a few seconds before orgasm, which will never allow release, and the pain of burning knives twisting in her genitals.

When self-effacing alters speak, they do not merely lack self-confidence; they are afraid to exist, and they think that they are the ugliest beings on earth. When kind and nurturing alters come out, they are not content to be kind to their friends or neighbors; they must save the planet. Whatever she experiences, in any personality, it is invariably the most intense form of that affect or state.

It is not enough that Bibi's mother abused her; she had the most abusive mother who has ever lived. Any positive qualities of Bibi's mother only prove how painful it is to have had a loving mother abuse you—much worse than a totally bad mother. The sexual abuse from her father was the worst anyone could have experienced.

Not surprisingly, Bibi's family members are extremely reserved in their expressed emotion, except during their own dissociative episodes, when emotion flows excessively. The only way to get noticed in her family was to be extreme. Bibi's symptoms began in first grade, but no one noticed. As a high school student, she had to get below 80 pounds for anyone to notice she was losing weight. As a college student, she had to get over 160 pounds for anyone to notice she was gaining.

Bibi had to tell a unique satanic story as well. Her satanists were of two varieties. One group wore white robes with velvet stripes, which she said looked Shakespearean in style. The other wore the usual black robes. The first group had their rituals in a secret amphitheater cut deep in the ground behind a famous public park. The second group tortured animals, killed people, and made the children eat raw body organs. Bibi was not content to have one kind of satanic abuse; she needed to have two.

Like Randi in Case 1, Bibi turns to her satanic material whenever we look closely at what happened with her mother and father. As treatment has progressed, the flamboyant and hyperbolic manner of expression has declined. She is undergoing the process of alters feeling each other's affects, and with that, the overall affective intensity is deepening while simultaneously becoming less exaggerated. At this time, she is beginning to wonder whether the satanic material is a distraction and an exaggeration—two concepts that were not part of her thinking before this therapy. Although it is too early to say for sure, the satanic aspects of Bibi's story seem to derive from deep characterological issues that cut across all the alters. She is beginning to discover that the events in her immediate family are more than sufficient to account for her symptoms and to ensure my interest and my help.

Discussion

Five cases present four prototypes of how satanic material can be used in therapy of MPD. Case 1 illustrates the use of satanic material as a projection and displacement of the knowledge and affect surrounding immediate family abuse. Of course, it is always theoretically possible that true satanic experiences were ignored in our work and disappeared not because they were primarily metaphors, but because they could be concealed by stories about father and mother. It is a theoretical possibility that no abuse emanated from Randi's parents and that the parent material was a disguise for the satanic. However, that possibility reflects the epistemological problem of proving the negative. From a clinical perspective, Randi continued to suffer her dissociation and her body memories while focusing on the satanic, and she moved toward integration and symptomatic relief when the therapy focused on the abuse within her immediate family. Although this explanation falls short of the logical proof one might want, it is compelling evidence that at least in some cases satanic memories serve as a displacement of family experiences that the patient needs to project and dissociate.

Case 2 illustrates the difficulty of distinguishing the true false-positive from the pseudofalse-positive MPD patient. MPD does not generally present in the flamboyant manner Patricia presented. Usually, an overblown presentation suggests that the diagnosis is not accurate. Patricia had heard that MPD was thought by some therapists to be linked to satanic experiences. How would her treatment have unfolded had she seen a therapist with an a priori disposition to regard satanic ritual cult abuse as a sine qua non of MPD?

Cases 3 and 4 demonstrate that not everything that swims is a fish. Sometimes experiences of group abuse are not satanic, or ritualistic, or cultic. However, there is a prevailing metaphoric vocabulary for describing group abuse, which some patients might use in the early phases of discovering their history. A wise therapist should reserve judgment and avoid leading patients toward a specific conclusion about the nature of the group that may have abused them.

Case 5 makes several points. The overall character structure of MPD patients is generally overlooked, yet MPD patients can have an overall structure just as patients with a single personality disorder can. Bibi revealed the dramatic, hyperbolic, intense, passionate character type we used to call "hysterical." In her case, these qualities suffused nearly all her alters. She had to be the most complex and difficult MPD patient there ever was, and she had not one, but two different kinds of satanic abuse stories.

I have long made the point that trauma, conflict, and deficiency all play a role in MPD and that our field today emphasizes trauma to the exclusion of other factors (Marmer 1991). Bibi illustrates that conflict and deficiency can shape character and can govern the unfolding of the treatment. Having MPD does not immunize a patient against character disorders, nor does it render a patient incapable of exaggeration or hyperbole. We have learned that where there's smoke, there's fire: where there is MPD, there is a strong probability of a history of childhood trauma. We have learned that many stories about trauma are based on fact, even if each and every detail of the patient's story might not be based on fact, even if each and every detail of the patient's story might not be exactly accurate. However, Bibi reminds us that MPD patients are fully capable of using their flashbacks for the same range of psychodynamic reasons that patients with a single personality disorder use their symptoms. Taking a patient's story at face value can be as serious a mistake as taking it solely as fantasy. The empathic stance of readiness to believe should not be incompatible with the necessity to interpret, and to distinguish, veridical memory from narrative or metaphoric memory.

Conclusion

I call myself a credulous skeptic because my approach embodies both parts of that apparent oxymoron. In the therapeutic alliance, I am ready to believe anything and everything, while also reserving skepticism about all. I try to hold this attitude in balance throughout the therapy. If I find myself surprised about a development toward the middle or end of therapy, I count this as a good sign.

With respect to satanic ritual cult abuse, the oxymoron applies even more strongly. The absence of hard evidence, the lack of this satanic material in my pre-1987 cases, and the stereotyping of so many elements of the stories patients tell about satanic material strengthen my skepticism. So too does the use of satanic material in a defensive way or for purpose of metaphor. The zeal of proponents in the debate over satanic ritual cult abuse likewise increases my skepticism.

On the other hand, I am credulous too. I could be persuaded to believe that satanic ritual cult abuse exists if the data came in. A number of years ago I called for the most sober and unsentimental scientists to test this issue (Marmer 1988). A modest and low-keyed confirmation would be much more convincing than a frantic and zealous one.

While stuck in my credulous skepticism, I have reported five anecdotes of patients who demonstrated at least four ways in which reports of satanic ritual cult abuse were dynamically important metaphors. With this in mind, perhaps more practitioners in the field of MPD and trauma could mix their therapeutic credulity with an appropriate amount of skepticism.

References

Freud S: The interpretation of dreams (1900), in The Standard Edition of the Complete Psychological Works of Sigmund Freud, Vols 4 and 5. Translated and edited by Strachey J. London, Hogarth Press, 1953

Freud S: Psycho-analytic notes on an autobiographical account of a case of paranoia (dementia paranoides) (1911), in The Standard Edition of the Complete Psychological Works of Sigmund Freud, Vol 12. Translated and edited by Strachey J. London, Hogarth Press, 1958, pp 1–82

Kluft RP: Clinical presentations of multiple personality disorder. Psychiatr
    Clin North Am 14:605–629, 1991
Marmer S: Whither MPD? comments on the state of the art in dissociation.
    Paper presented at the Sixth International Conference on Multiple
    Personality/Dissociative States, Chicago, IL, October 1988
Marmer S: Multiple personality disorder: a psychoanalytic perspective.
    Psychiatr Clin North Am 14:677–694, 1991
Masson J: The Assault on the Truth. New York, Farrar, Straus & Giroux,
    1984
Niederland WG: The Schreber Case. New York, Quadrangle/The New
    York Times Book Co, 1974
Schafer R: The Analytic Attitude. New York, Basic Books, 1983
Spence DP: Narrative Truth and Historical Truth: Meaning and Interpre-
    tation in Psychoanalysis. New York, WW Norton, 1982

CHAPTER 2

Hypnosis and Memory: A Cautionary Chapter

Joseph Barber, Ph.D.

We know that the trusting, benevolent alliance developed between psychotherapist and patient is paramount to the success of psychotherapy. Essential to this alliance is the patient's experiencing the therapist as believing in the patient and validating the patient's experiences. However, does this validation require that we actually believe as factual the experiences reported by the patient? If a patient whom we know to be schizophrenic reports that he or she hears voices, we are likely to believe that the report is truthful, even though we do not believe that living persons actually are speaking to the patient. If a paranoid patient reports that someone is out to get him or her, we take as factual his or her experience and belief of this threat, without necessarily believing that someone is actually intending harm to the patient.

The clinician faces a dilemma, however, when the experience reported by the patient may require action. If the schizophrenic patient reports that the voices are commanding him or her to harm someone, and the patient intends to do harm, it is not sufficient that we merely believe in the patient's experience of harmfulness; we are required to take action to prevent that harm from occurring.

I am grateful to Mary Pepping, Ph.D., for her insightful comments on the ideas expressed in this chapter.

If a child reports being abused, it is not sufficient that we merely offer sympathy to the child; we are required to take action to protect the child from further abuse, recognizing that this protection outweighs the risk of harm to the child and to the family.

In certain instances, a clinician must confront the reliability of the patient's report. If the patient reports that he or she intends to do harm to someone, we must assess the seriousness and reality of that intent. If the patient is merely expressing a fantasy or a desire, with no real intent to carry it out, good clinical practice requires that we take no action to protect the would-be victim. If the child's report is merely a report of fantasy or confabulation, good clinical practice requires that we take no action to protect the child.

Pertinent to this book, if a patient, adult or child, reports having been abused in a ritualistic fashion, what should we do? How does a clinician assess the veracity of a patient's report? When a patient reports the experience of a dream, we take the experience seriously, but we do not assume that the events of the dream actually occurred. When a patient reports an experience as fantasy, we do not assume the fantasy parallels actual life events (although, of course, we might, in certain circumstances, take such primary process reports as evidence of some parallel in the patient's life). How do we distinguish historical fact from narrative fiction, conscious or unconscious, intended or unwitting?

Further complicating the issue is the nature of the victims of abuse. Although adult men are sometimes victims, it is far more often the case that victims of abuse are women and children. Historically, women and children reporting a history of sexual abuse were not taken seriously; rather, their claims have sometimes been interpreted as fantasy. The contemporary struggle for enlightenment with respect to equal treatment of women and humane treatment of children evokes an almost reflexive inclination to believe a woman's or a child's claims of abuse, no matter what the evidence, as an understandable attempt to counter the long-standing inclination not to take them seriously, no matter what the evidence.

Throughout history, civilizations have sought means to discover the truth underlying an individual's testimony. Although we no longer trust in a priest's or shaman's methods, contemporary society still longs for a means of uncovering the truth. Our current means involve methods that seem to carry scientific probability. The premier examples of truth serum in our culture are hypnosis and Sodium Amytal. In this chapter, I evaluate evidence for the qualities of hypnosis as truth serum. I also summarize the best current understanding of the reliability of memory. Finally, I offer suggestions to the clinician faced with the patient whose reports of abuse must be assessed and treated.

The Fallibility of Hypnosis

No single definition of hypnosis is universally accepted (Hilgard 1991). To clarify what is meant by hypnosis in this chapter, the following description is useful:

> Hypnosis is an altered state of consciousness in which the individual's imagination creates vivid reality from suggestions offered either by someone else, by suggestions inferred from environmental cues, or by suggestions initiated by the individual himself or herself. This condition allows the individual to be inordinately responsive to such suggestions, so that he or she is able to alter perception, memory and physiological processes that under ordinary conditions are not readily susceptible to conscious control. (Barber 1992, p. 244)

Two of the characteristics referred to in this description are especially pertinent to the discussion of hypnosis in this chapter: the capacity to create vivid reality from suggestions and the capacity to alter memory. These capacities are examined, beginning with the issue of memory.

Since the beginning of this century, it has been widely believed that hypnosis enhances an individual's capacity for accurate recall. However, systematic investigation of the issue reveals that this belief is incorrect. Although there are anecdotal accounts of the value of hypnosis in uncovering forgotten information (Kroger and Douce 1979), such accounts seem exceptional. Stalnaker and Riddle's (1932) report made clear that hypnotized subjects' recall of literary selections learned in a prior year could be improved by the use of hypnosis. However, their improvement in recall was confounded by inclusion of inaccurate memory. Without independent verification, it would not have been possible to determine that some of their improved memory contained substantial inaccuracy. Fifty years later, Dywan and Bowers (1983) reported, similarly, that hypnotized university students improved their memory of items on a word list, but they also recalled a substantial number of words not on the list.

Whether or not an individual correctly recalls words on a list does not necessarily reflect memory capacity in daily life. Unfortunately, this disconcerting finding is not limited to the context of the laboratory. The forensic application of hypnosis has had a stormy history. Can an individual's recall of a crime or other trauma be refreshed by hypnotic suggestion? Orne et al. (1988) reported a significant number of forensic cases in which hypnotized witnesses testified to remembering seeing events that were physically impossible to have seen and to a variety of other demonstrably false facts. Although these memory distortions were presumably innocently created, subtle cuing of hypnotized subjects can produce profoundly believed-in but totally false memory.

Not only the distortion of memory is at issue, but also the complete and honest certainty with which individuals report the distortions. Because it is such certainty in the accuracy of one's own memory that supports the credibility of completely mistaken forensic witnesses, the application of hypnosis in forensic circumstances is a very hazardous undertaking. Although reports such as that of Kroger and Douce (1979) seem to suggest that hypnosis sometimes can produce accurate memories, this can be determined only with the aid of independent verification. This issue has become clarified in recent years in the forensic context, and the courts have taken these facts into appropriate consideration. However, although the same capacities for memory distortion can be obtained in the clinical context, clinicians generally seem opaque to the problem.

When a hypnotized patient reports an experience, the usual response of the clinician is to believe the patient's report as if it is historically true. However, the danger of misinterpreting a patient's hypnotized reports cannot be overemphasized. The competent clinician must keep in mind that the likelihood of a patient developing a distorted memory while hypnotized—of confidently recalling images, feelings, thoughts, perceptions, and other experiences that are at least partly, and perhaps totally, the result of imagination—is an ever-present factor.

Hypnosis does not necessarily improve the accuracy of a patient's memory. It is likely that a hypnotized patient will unwittingly imagine events yet believe the imagined experience to be historically accurate.

A clinician must remember that what a hypnotized patient reports may be completely accurate, may be partly accurate and partly imagined, or may be completely imagined. In the absence of independent means of verification, there is no known means of determining the truth of a patient's reports, whether the patient is hypnotized or not. Many clinicians believe that they can tell whether or not a patient is telling the truth; however, there is no evidence to support such a conceit. It must be remembered that the issue is not whether the patient is telling the truth or lying. The assumption underlying this discussion is that the patient is conscientiously attempting to be truthful and accurate in reporting. Such an attempt, however, is no match for the power of the human imagination, hypnotized or not.

The other characteristic of hypnosis is the capacity to create vivid reality from imagination. A nocturnal dream is ordinarily the occasion for the believed-in reality of a completely imagined experience. The experience imagery also is laden with affect, and probably laden with psychological import. This imagery, because it is weighted with meaning and affect, has an important use in psychotherapy. However, just as a nocturnal dream is generally interpreted as a metaphor by the clinician—not taken as a journalistic account of the patient's life—any report from the patient, nocturnal or otherwise, hypnotically induced or otherwise, also must be interpreted as a metaphor.

For example, a patient may have symptoms of depression and interpersonal difficulties. Perhaps avoidance of sexual and other intimate contact is an issue. Suppose that hypnosis is incorporated in the therapy—perhaps to promote a more comfortable, trusting attitude toward the clinician. Suppose, further, that the patient begins to report images of physical and sexual abuse. As the patient reports these images, the patient also experiences appropriately disturbed affect in response to these images. What is the clinician to make of these reports? Is there any reason to believe that these images reflect historically accurate events in the patient's life? Symptoms of depression and interpersonal difficulties are recognizably associated with abusive histories. But there are other etiologies for these symptoms as well.

Frankel's (1993) review of reported childhood events in the multiple personality literature clearly suggests the rarity with which a patient's history, including claims of abuse, is ever independently documented. Although this lack of documentation may be understandable, given the difficulties, logistic and otherwise, in trying to document an adult's childhood history, the fact also should give us pause for two reasons.

First, individuals who are unhappy are necessarily seeking a reason for their unhappiness. Even if they had no prior memory of childhood abuse, nor reason to suspect abuse, the current widespread cultural emphasis on childhood abuse as the primary underlying source of adult unhappiness provides at least the question, in many people's minds, about their own childhood histories. In addition to the ubiquity of childhood abuse in the media, a virtual specialty market within psychotherapy has developed to assess and treat this problem. Books feature clinicians who claim childhood abuse as the primary source of a myriad of neurotic symptomatology (Bass and Davis 1988).

Second, although anyone is potentially susceptible to suggestion from such an affect-charged cultural environment, some individuals' susceptibility to suggestion is quite high. Patients carrying the diagnosis of multiple personality disorder, for example, also tend to have unusually high hypnotic responsivity (Frankel 1993). Other patients, even those whose disorders are far less severe, can be characterized by such responsivity. It is quite possible, then, for an unhappy person, pondering the source of his or her unhappiness, to begin unwittingly to generate images, feelings, and thoughts, which he or she also interprets as recall of actual experience—even though the images, feelings, and thoughts are being generated for the first time. Yet this person, supported by the current cultural climate, has no reason to consider the possibility that these experiences are imagined; rather, he or she is supported by a variety of sources in the interpretation that the experiences are sudden, derepressed memories of earlier traumatic events. If the person's clinician is also a source for this interpretation, a fully realized and totally erroneous belief about a traumatic experience is likely to develop.

The Fallibility of Memory

When recall occurs in the clinical situation, either through hypnosis or other nonhypnotic means, the pressure to interpret the experience as fact rather than fantasy becomes compelling—particularly when the clinician naively assumes that anything a patient manifests must be true. "Why would someone make this up?" is a question I've often heard in the context of clinicians discussing this issue. Yet this question is asked in apparent ignorance of a substantial literature that explains why, indeed, someone "makes this up" (e.g., Loftus 1982, 1993).

Although it remains to be demonstrated that findings from affectively neutral laboratory memory research can be generalized to the clinical world of trauma, the considerable body of research done by Loftus (1993) and other scientists who study human memory processes effectively demonstrates that the attractive tape-recorder model of memory is inaccurate. This appealingly simple model has been replaced by a less appealing one—for those of us who wish to be confident in the reliability of memory. The contemporary model describes memory as a highly complex, constantly evolving process, always susceptible to alteration by the individual's psychological needs. It should be noted that this model has been developed from laboratory studies not obviously related to the affect-charged memories reported by clinical patients. However, in the absence of contradictory evidence, this empirically based model certainly suggests the need for caution in the way a clinician interprets a patient's report of memory.

For some people, there is reason to believe that repressed memories have lain silent for years, suddenly to erupt with full-blown accuracy. However, there is little scientific evidence supporting reliability of the increasingly widespread reports of sudden recovery of memories of early trauma (Loftus 1993). In the absence of independent verification of adult reconstruction of childhood events, what evidence does the clinician have to determine the historical accuracy of a patient's report? Most often, clinicians interpret the processing, the working through, of such memories during the course of psychotherapy and the subsequent resolution of symptoms as proof that the reports were accurate. Although this criterion is appealing, and seems to be supported by a kind of intuitive reasoning, closer examination suggests its inadequacy. Wright (1993a) describes the case, familiar to many psychotherapists, of a patient who presented with anxiety symptoms, which he believed to be the result of abduction by beings from another planet. Following psychotherapeutic treatment, the anxiety symptoms came under control: the cured patient left therapy, believing that he was once abducted by aliens.

This case is similar to those of patients who present for treatment with the belief that traumatic events in a past life are responsible for current symptomatology. I once treated a woman who had a phobia of blood and who believed the intense anxiety symptoms were a result of a long-forgotten childhood trauma. Using hypnotic age regression, we explored her childhood memories, none of which seemed to be sufficient to account for the intensity of her symptoms. I then suggested to her that she develop an even deeper state of hypnosis so that, if a forgotten event were responsible for her current condition, she might be able to remember it. After a period of quiescence, during which I assumed she was experiencing deep reflection, she began to manifest an unexpected and very intense abreaction, culminating in an exceedingly dramatic report of trauma experienced in the nineteenth-century Irish Civil War. Although I did not believe this young woman had actually been present during that century-old conflict, I nonetheless took her experience seriously and facilitated the working through of the affect associated with this experience. In the minutes following the hypnotic experience, she seemed to be free of any anxiety about blood. Seven years later, during a serendipitous meeting, she revealed that she had remained free of the anxiety symptoms. Although I cannot prove that a patient was not really affected by events in a past life, and cannot prove that another was not abducted by aliens, I do not personally believe in the reality of these claims. Until future events prove otherwise, I prefer a more parsimonious hypothesis: humans have a powerful capacity to make emotionally meaningful fantasy experiences seem totally, believably real.

The successful use of imagination in psychotherapy is ubiquitous—notably in psychodrama, or gestalt therapy, or psychoanalysis—but present in all therapy, even the most basic behavior therapies. If the imagination of the underlying cause of a symptom has personal meaning to the patient, would we not predict the therapeutic usefulness of this imagination, accurate or not? However, the efficacy of its use cannot be taken as evidence of the veracity of the imagined experience. Or, of course, in the absence of independent verification, can we know if the imagined experience is not true? The simple if disconcerting truth is we *cannot* know.

Some years ago, I described the case of a man suffering from a dramatic form of dyssomnia (Barber 1986). During the course of treatment involving hypnotically induced nocturnal dream recall, this man began to report the recall of traumatic childhood events. Also during treatment, which included working through of the thoughts and feelings associated with these memories, the symptoms of dyssomnia began to abate. I had no way to verify the reality of the traumatic events described by that patient. I tended to believe they were accurately recalled, although I have no way to know if this is so. Perhaps they were largely the product of the patient's imagination. Fortunately, in this case, I did not need to know. The resolution of the symptoms was sufficient for the patient to be satisfied. This case occurred in the late 1970s. In the current climate, however, as increasingly happens, such a patient might well seek legal recourse against the perpetrator of these childhood traumas. And what defense can be offered, after so many years? It becomes simply an issue of the plaintiff's word against the defendant's.

Wright (1993a, 1993b) describes the recent case of adolescent daughters' claims that they were the victims of satanic ritual abuse. Their father's subsequent criminal conviction and imprisonment for this criminal abuse occurred in the absence of any evidence whatsoever for the existence of the crime. As a consequence of society's current emphasis on abuse victims' rights, believing victims' claims of abuse, and punishing the perpetrators of abuse, there is a growing vulnerability to creating victims of the falsely accused (Loftus and Ketcham 1991). One of the challenges to a just society is maintaining the difficult balance between prosecuting the crimes against victims and defending the rights of the accused. A crucial element in that balance is the proper understanding of the nature of memory and the dismaying degree of the fallibility of memory.

Also as a consequence of society's current emphasis on abuse victims' rights, it becomes crucially important to keep in mind that a report obtained in the context of psychotherapy has no greater likelihood of being historically accurate and reliable than any other claim. This is true whether or not hypnosis was used in the reporting of the history. The report may be an accurate reflection of historical events, or it may contain a kernel of truth, elaborated by psychologically meaningful metaphor. Or, the report may be wholly an unconscious result of an adult's need to find some attribution for his or her unhappiness. Quite often, using a seemingly commonsensical approach, a clinician relies on the patient's confidence in the report, and the specificity of its detail, as a criterion for determining its veracity. However, it must be remembered that the conviction with which the patient reports the memories, and even the specificity of detail with which they are described, is totally unrelated to their accuracy.

The Problem

We all know the seemingly limitless human capacity for harming one another. There is demonstrable evidence of the grotesque abuse that is done, primarily by men, to women and children. I recognize that questioning the reliability of a patient's report of abuse risks the perception by some that I am unsympathetic to and ignorant of the gravity of the problem of physical and sexual abuse. However, nothing in this chapter is intended to deny the terrible daily reality of physical and sexual abuse.

The fact that abuse occurs does not indicate that every report of abuse is an accurate one. However, clinicians' misguided reliance on the archaic tape-recorder model of memory and their uninformed belief in the truth-serum quality of hypnosis create a further permutation of the problem of abuse. An uncritical, credulous acceptance of any and all claims of abuse has, on its own, serious and harmful consequences.

The secondary level of abuse perpetrated against parents wrongly accused is sufficiently tragic to claim our attention. Another harmful consequence of therapists' naive credulity in patients' claims of childhood abuse is the increasingly strident cultural backlash against the whole enterprise of psychotherapy. The False Memory Syndrome Foundation has developed a response to this social problem. One might wish that the primary target of hostility by this group, an increasingly powerful voice in the community, would be the abuse of children by parents. Unfortunately, the target is psychotherapy itself. Many members of this group perceive psychotherapists to be the primary cause of the problem, engaging in the reckless ruination of families. This perception is sometimes correct. Clearly, it is crucially important for clinicians to become knowledgeable about the issues of abuse, to know that the truth of a patient's claim is impossible to determine, and to avoid unwittingly creating a patient's experience of abuse out of the psychotherapeutic process.

Suggestions for Clinicians

How should a clinician respond to a patient who produces nocturnal dreams or images during therapy or uncovers memories that might suggest a history of traumatic abuse?

First, of course, it is important that any clinician be aware of the possibility of countertransference in his or her approach to the patient. If a clinician has unresolved feelings about abuse, either personal or otherwise, it is natural that these feelings will exert pressure, perhaps unconsciously, to interpret the patient's symptoms or reports in the context of abuse. As in any therapeutic circumstance, it is important that a clinician make effective use of supervision resources. The pursuit of personal therapy to become aware of unresolved feelings and to find means to their successful resolution is critical to adequate conduct as a clinician. How many psychotherapists have had sufficient psychotherapy themselves? How many are sufficiently clear about their own coun-tertransferential processes?

Second, the context of psychotherapy itself inclines clinicians toward searching for a history of trauma as a source for contempo-rary troubles. Although this search for history is a necessary and appropriate part of psychotherapy, we need to be alert to its haz-ards. The possibility of confirmatory bias—the tendency for thera-pists to search for reasons to confirm (and not to disconfirm) personal hypotheses—makes us vulnerable to particular interpre-tations (Baron et al. 1988).

Third, it is important that the clinician recognize the possibil-ity of memory contamination in the process of treatment. It is essential for a clinician to be aware of, and contain, his or her personal beliefs about a patient's history and to keep those be-liefs from influencing the therapeutic environment. For exam-ple, leading questions, comments about abuse, and intensity of response to a patient's reports can all contribute to the unwitting creation of a patient's memory, including memory of traumatic abuse. It can be quite difficult to remain open, without finding a resolution, to the question of the veracity of a patient's reports. However, in the absence of independent evidence, there is no way to determine such veracity. Unless there is a way to verify independently a patient's history, the clinician must be willing to remain open to all possibilities. It may be that the patient was abused, and it may be that the patient was not abused. There is no way to know. This is a fact that the patient needs to accept as well. It can sometimes be clinically challenging to be both empa-thetic to the patient and open to the interpretation of the pa-tient's experiences. But, of course, this challenge is always a central part of the enterprise of psychotherapy. Fortunately, it is not necessary for a clinician to develop a credulous attitude about a patient's reports in order to facilitate healing.

As clinicians, we need to be vigilant about the degree of caution required in handling cases where there is a possibility of traumatic abuse. I hope I have conveyed my own anxiety, concern, and em-pathy about the difficulty of contending with these issues. A certain amount of wariness about one's capacity to deal with these cases suggests, I think, a salutary degree of good clinical judgment.

References

Barber J: The case of Superman: integrating hypnosis and gestalt therapy in the treatment of dyssomnia, in Case Studies in Hypnotherapy. Edited by Dowd E, Healy J. New York, Guilford, 1986, pp 46–60

Barber J: The locksmith model: accessing hypnotic responsiveness, in Theories of Hypnosis: Current Models and Perspectives. Edited by Lynn S, Rhue J. New York, Guilford, 1992, pp 241–274

Baron J, Beattie J, Hershey J: Heuristics and biases in diagnostic reasoning: congruence, information, and certainty. Organizational Behaviour and Human Decision Processes 42:88–110, 1988

Bass E, Davis L: The Courage to Heal. New York, Harper & Row, 1988

Dywan J, Bowers K: The use of hypnosis to enhance recall. Science 222:184–185, 1983

Frankel F: Adult reconstruction of childhood events in the multiple personality literature. Am J Psychiatry 150:954–958, 1993

Hilgard E: A neodissociation interpretation of hypnosis, in Theories of Hypnosis: Current Models and Perspectives. Edited by Lynn S, Rhue J. New York, Guilford, 1991, pp 83–104

Kroger W, Douce R: Hypnosis in criminal investigation. Int J Clin Exp Hypn 27:358–374, 1979

Loftus E: Memory and its distortions, in G. Stanley Hall Lectures. Edited by Kraut AG. Washington, DC, American Psychological Association, 1982, pp 119–154

Loftus E: The reality of repressed memories. Am Psychol 48:518–537, 1993

Loftus E, Ketcham K: Witness for the Defense. New York, St. Martin's Press, 1991

Orne M, Whitehouse W, Dinges D, et al: Reconstructing memory through hypnosis: forensic and clinical implications, in Hypnosis and Memory. Edited by Pettinati H. New York, Guilford, 1988, pp 21–54

Stalnaker J, Riddle F: The effect of hypnosis on long-delayed recall. J Gen Psychol 6:429–440, 1932

Wright L: Remembering Satan, part 1. The New Yorker, May 17, 1993a, pp 60–81

Wright L: Remembering Satan, part 2. The New Yorker, May 24, 1993b, pp 57–76

Overview of the Treatment of Patients Alleging That They Have Suffered Ritualized or Sadistic Abuse

Richard P. Kluft, M.D.

Ritualized abuse, satanic ritualized abuse, sadistic abuse, cult abuse, multivictim-multiperpetrator abuse—these are some of the many terms that have been proposed to describe a perplexing and thought-provoking phenomenon reported by an increasing number of deeply distressed individuals who have presented for treatment during the last decade. Primarily in these past 10 years, mental health professionals of all disciplines, most of whom have had no prior experience with such allegations, have found themselves confronted with patients who state that they have (or suspect that they have) experienced or participated in bizarre and outlandish ceremonies during which acts of sexual excess, brutality, mutilation, murder, human sacrifice, cannibalism, and consumption of foul substances were commonplace. Often these practices are said to be associated with homage to Satan or the celebration of some other worldview in which these or similar beliefs and behaviors play an intrinsic part.

A large number of the patients reporting such experiences have been given the diagnosis of multiple personality disorder (MPD), renamed dissociative identity disorder (DID) in DSM-IV (American Psychiatric Association 1994). As a rule, they have described themselves as the victims of other abuses as well, usually within their families. Often, these patients have alleged that their family members had participated in the ritualized abuse experiences as well.

Many clinicians and law enforcement officials were initially sympathetic to these accounts, made as they were in the context of the rise of feminism and enhanced societal sensitivity to the exploitation of women and children, with increasing professional and media attention being drawn to domestic violence, incest, rape, child abuse, sexual harassment, and numerous other injustices and abuses. They suspended the automatic disbelief that such extraordinary narratives might ordinarily inspire. American society, with psychotherapists in the vanguard, has become increasingly sensitive to the plight of the victim or survivor of malice or misfortune and ready to reconsider the long-neglected role of real trauma in the causation of psychopathology.

Although those who first embraced the reality of their patients' accounts of ritualized abuse encountered opposition, criticism, and derision among their colleagues, most persisted. It was easy to observe the rapid polarization of the two camps, each mistrustful and often derisive of the other. An uneasy atmosphere saturated with insults, innuendos, and ad hominem attacks developed and has persisted. Many organizations whose members were concerned with phenomena and issues pertinent to this debate found themselves divided by painful schisms.

Other constituencies were drawn into the maelstrom. Many victim or survivor groups—insisting that the memories of abused individuals were accurate, and sensitive to the disbelief too often encountered by those who protest their mistreatment—were inclined to endorse the accounts of those who alleged ritualized abuse at the hands of satanists. Numerous religious groups that explicitly accept the existence of Satan and demons, and perceive the world as a battleground between good and evil, found such allegations consistent with their belief systems and cosmologies. The rise of historical revisionism, especially with regard to denying the reality of the Holocaust, inspired many to bend over backward not to dismiss unfairly accounts of what might be a hidden Holocaust of serious proportions.

On the other hand, many clinicians and academicians had become increasingly concerned over what they believed was the overdiagnosis of MPD (DID), the overly credulous acceptance of allegations of child abuse, and the misuse of certain interviewing procedures (such as certain forms of questioning and hypnosis); they were readily recruited into or eagerly entered the ranks of those who doubted the reality of accounts of ritualized abuse. Many of these individuals pointed to the media's exploitation of sensationalistic materials, the possibility of contagion in peer-led or leaderless support groups, and the risk of iatrogenesis and confabulation in therapeutic settings.

Groups purporting to speak for those who claim to have been falsely accused of child abuse have found it useful to exploit the skepticism surrounding alleged ritualized abuse as a starting point for their efforts to demolish the credibility of those making more mundane accusations. Their strategy has seemed geared to finding a straw-man target and then initiating a domino effect that serves their agendas: first, they attack the credibility of allegations of ritualistic abuses, for which there is minimal documentation; then proceed to attack the credibility of MPD (DID), the disorder of most patients who make such allegations; then undermine the credibility of other accusations of abuse made by this now-discredited group; and then challenge the memories and allegations of virtually all individuals making accusations of abuse. In this manner, the credibility of those alleging childhood abuse, especially on the basis of recovering formerly repressed or dissociated memories, would be cast under a cloud of suspicion.

Patrons of both polarities not only disagreed, but many also behaved in a manner that initiated an era of nastiness and character assassination. For example, it was not uncommon for prominent persons who expressed a disbelief in cults and cult abuse to be accused of being cult related somehow, nor was it unusual for those who expressed a belief in ritualized abuse to lose their professional and personal credibility overnight. Those who took a moderate or agnostic stance often were assailed from both sides. I held and hold a moderate point of view and routinely encounter disparagement from enthusiasts representing both polarities when I lecture on the subject.

Personal Reflections

My own perspective follows naturally from my clinical experiences and from my reading and learning. Early in my training, I was made aware of the problematic nature of memory in general and of recollections facilitated by hypnosis in particular. Both my psychoanalytically oriented preceptors and my teachers in the field of hypnosis made it clear that fantasy, context (including demand characteristics), and suggestion, however subtle, could impel a patient to report as a memory an event or events that had never occurred or had occurred differently from the scenarios that had been reported to me.

Therefore, when I first interviewed the alleged abusers of one of my first MPD (DID) patients, I was fully prepared to hear them disconfirm what their daughter had reported in the context of therapy, both in her baseline accounts of her past and in what she had recalled in the process of treatment, from both psychoanalytic psychotherapy and sessions involving hypnosis. I was flabbergasted to find that they confirmed her accounts in all major details. Later in my work with the same patient, I was able to find some memories that could be definitively disconfirmed, despite the fact that they retained their compelling sense of reality to the patient and had been recounted in great detail with intense affect and apparently sincere conviction. Such experiences caused me to observe that "in a given patient, one may find episodes of photographic recall, confabulation, screen phenomena, confusion between dreams or fantasies and reality, irregular recollection, and wilful misrepresentation. One awaits goodness of fit among several forms of data, and often must be satisfied to remain uncertain" (Kluft 1984, p. 14).

My first experience with ritualized abuse allegations also occurred in the mid-1970s, long before the current spate of reports. An MPD (DID) patient was referred to me for consultation and possible treatment. The referring clinician said she could not resolve a conflict among the patient's alters over whether the patient would continue to attend nocturnal satanic gatherings. The patient was a woman in her thirties attending a small college. Her problem had first been revealed to a male professor, who had referred her for treatment. He remained quite concerned about his student, in whom he took a particular interest.

Although the woman declined to return for appointments after evaluation, for a time the therapist, the professor, and I remained in contact, hoping she could be persuaded to enter treatment. Without sharing his plans, the professor followed her on nights he suspected she might be involved in satanic activity. After some unsuccessful efforts, he was able to drive after her, unobserved, to a remote wooded area. He followed her into the woods but lost her in the dark. In the course of his search, he saw a bonfire in the distance. He drew near and observed a number of people changing into dark robes around the fire. He was noticed and driven off with blows, kicks, and curses. As he looked back, he saw the people smother the fire rapidly and disperse. He shared this with me the following morning. I saw no reason to doubt this account, which suggests much and confirms little.

Over the next several years, I began to hear increasingly frequent accounts of organized satanic cults from patients with MPD (DID), several of whom maintained that they were still participating in cult activities. Some behaved as if they were still involved. In one case, a patient indicated she was about to sacrifice her young child, who she claimed had been conceived during an orgiastic satanic ritual. Police surveillance determined that she was in fact going to a remote wooded area on nights she claimed to be involved in cult activities, but the officers did not succeed in following her to her final destination. I was moved to involve child protective authorities because although I could not be sure that my patient was in fact involved with a cult, I could be sure that she was very disturbed and had repeatedly stated in detail her plans to kill her child (Kluft 1987). I also encountered a great number of instances in which patients mentioned very unique details and those details would be mentioned years later by another patient with whom there was no evidence of interim contact or any contact at all.

Notwithstanding the impressions created by these incidents, other experiences occurring at the same time suggested yet another perspective. I had decided to keep records of all alleged cult-related murders, kidnappings, and sacrifices reported by my patients and those I saw in consultation. After a few years, it became apparent that if my patients' accounts were accurate, they would have depopulated the counties in which they lived. Clearly, either wholesale slaughter was occurring without perceptible impact or most if not all of the killing simply had not taken place. Although patients often took pains to stress the cleverness of the cult in concealing all traces of its activities, it was difficult to accept as plausible that such decimating carnage, involving so many victims and perpetrators, had left no conclusive evidence of its occurrence.

I had the further experience of receiving repeated threats on my life. For example, on many occasions during a 2-month period when I answered my telephone personally, a deep voice would say that I was getting too close to cult secrets and would be killed if I did not back off. Although these telephone calls were extremely disquieting, after a brief period of serious concern I sensed a pattern in them. I confronted the patient I suspected was either making or instigating the calls. Although I got no admission or confirmation, I never received another threatening call.

I also found that some patients brought up cultic material whenever certain dynamics were at play in the therapy and that others' allegations were not unusual but disquietingly impossible. On other occasions, I was able to find that some personalities were claiming credit for making other alters believe that they were involved with or in danger from individuals associated with ritual abuse activities. On one occasion, an inpatient reported that she was receiving telephone messages from the cult instructing her to kill one of my colleagues and/or me. She assured me she would commit suicide rather than kill another. I arranged for the patient to be kept away from the telephone for a few days without the patient being aware of this intent. She continued to report receiving calls from the cult. When confronted gently, she initially denied the calls, and finally an alter confessed that it had the capacity to convince other alters that events had occurred by creating compellingly vivid hallucinatory occurrences.

I hope that this summary conveys some notion of the nature of the clinical encounters to which I was exposed and which left me very respectful of their diversity and complexity. My craving for a simplistic and reassuring understanding has remained frustrated, and I remain a moderate, or agnostic, with respect to the reality of ritualized abuse. More often than not, the data available to me as a clinician simply do not allow me to determine whether a given allegation is accurate or erroneous. It is my best judgment that alternative explanations are plausible for the majority of the allegations of ritual abuse to which I have been exposed, but those alternatives do not account unequivocally for every report.

Heuristic Approaches Explaining Ritualistic Abuse

Current heuristic approaches that explain alleged ritualistic abuse are as follows:

1. *Many if not all of the allegations are accurate depictions of historical reality.* A number of authorities endorse the likelihood of the reality of allegations of satanic ritual abuse. The works of Smith and Pazder (1980), whose book *Michelle Remembers* is often cited as a key document in the field, and Friesen (1991), author of *Uncovering the Mystery of MPD*, exemplify this literature. Many publications with this affirmative perspective are saturated with religious overtones; beliefs are frequently accorded the stature of facts. Although many voices have been raised protesting the mental health consequences of promulgating a worldview conducive to spreading distress about matters satanic, it is difficult for the psychotherapist to deal with the unfortunate consequences of a religion's belief system. Another subset of proponents cite apparent historical evidences for the persistence of deviant groups over time (e.g., Hill and Goodwin 1989, who are not associated with this view but whose paper is often cited in its defense). This stance is countered by those who point to the dearth of objective evidence for such phenomena.
2. *No evidence exists to prove the reality of such allegations, necessitating alternative hypotheses in all cases.* Lanning (1991), from the law enforcement perspective, Putnam (1991), and Ganaway (1989, 1990) have put forward this hypothesis, pointing out that the dearth of hard evidence despite thousands of allegations of ritualistic abuse makes it very unlikely that they are substantial. These arguments are countered by those attributing great ingenuity to the cult in covering its tracks.

3. *A syndrome exists in which such allegations are made, and that syndrome deserves our serious study.* This heuristic perspective has been offered by Young et al. (1991) in their study of the phenomenology of a series of patients alleging ritual abuse experiences. These researchers are agnostic with respect to belief and argue that the study of the syndrome will ultimately lead to better understanding of its etiology. Related to this hypothesis are attempts to conceptualize accounts of ritual abuse as a variety of Munchausen syndrome (Goodwin 1988; Ross 1995).

4. *Ritualistic abuse groups exist, but their actual behavior is other than what is reported by patients.* According to this perspective, groups induce their victims to believe that horrific events have occurred. However, most if not all of the events are illusory, and the patient's perception of them is affected by the clever manipulation of hypnosis, mind-altering drugs, misdirection and the creation of illusion, and other tools of thought control rather than by witnessing and participating in actual atrocities (R. J. Loewenstein, personal communications, March 1989– October 1991). Ganaway (1989) has addressed some aspects of this hypothesis.

5. *Therapists overtly and covertly provoke their patients to create such accounts.* This position is widely believed by skeptics of ritual abuse allegations. Skeptics hold that both by pressuring patients with inappropriately leading and insinuating questions and by creating an atmosphere in which differential attention is paid to such allegations, the therapist induces the patient to initiate, continue, and believe in the reality of satanic ritual abuse. Therapists themselves give credence to accounts of ritualized abuse by virtue of credulity, religious orientations that endorse the reality of satanic agency, and training environments that, whether deliberately or covertly, induce them to believe in the actuality of these accounts. Mulhern (1991) describes treatments in which beliefs in ritualized abuse are accepted and in which evidence of ritualized abuse involvement is avidly pursued as "cultified therapy" (p. 158). She argues that a "belief filter" is created by training and expectation such that "paranoid interpretation" is applied to clinical data:

> Fortuitous illusory similarities [between clinical data and cult-credulous beliefs and observations] are made to appear relevant because they are viewed through a belief filter that overestimates coincidences that can be explained in other ways. . . . In other words, *the alleged victims of satanic cults are not so much saying the same things as they are being heard in the same way.* (Mulhern 1991, p. 158, brackets and italics in original)

Thus, satanism, like beauty, is in the eyes of the beholder. This perspective is valuable in understanding the situation of the believing therapist but does not explain the emergence of accounts of satanic ritual abuse in the caseload of the scrupulously agnostic or skeptical therapist.

6. *Patients bring to therapy ego contents that are imbued with a belief in ritualized abuse.* Greaves (1992) has done an excellent analysis of the possible mechanisms involved in creating this belief. In the *incorporation hypothesis*, the patient has unconsciously internalized information that is falsely remembered as his or her own, a form of source amnesia. Although there are many materials from which a patient might learn a cultic view of the world and the hypothesis is attractive, Greaves notes that 1) contact with such sources is routinely denied by patients, 2) he never has encountered a patient whose account parallels available sources, and 3) systematic and prolonged study would be necessary to absorb the materials with which allegers seem familiar.

The *screen memory hypothesis* holds that real or fantasied memories disguise a deeper conflict. Ganaway (1989), Van Benschoten (1990), and Noll (1992) have discussed this hypothesis. Greaves (1992), however, wonders if this idea can be sustained because the overall memory bank of the patient alleging experiences of ritualistic abuse is replete with all sorts of horror, so the idea that something worse is being hidden is hard to sustain. Later in this chapter, I argue that certain more mundane abuses actually may be worse psychological blows because they involve the loss of hope for parental love. For many, these mundane experiences can prove to be a more devastating psychological trauma than exposure to horrific experiences.

The *urban legend hypothesis* holds that patients pick up the idea of satanic cults from urban legends, which are tales told first as a joke or prank and then spread by gossip by those who want to perpetuate the hoax and those who believe it to be genuine. A typical example concerns the notion that the sewers of New York are full of alligators descended from tiny alligators brought home as souvenirs of Florida years ago and flushed down the toilet when they were no longer of interest to their owners. Although subscribing to this hypothesis is tempting, accounts of ritualistic abuse differ from typical urban legends in many crucial respects, including point of view (first person rather than hearsay), affective charge, protestations of proof, elaborateness, failure to circulate in the general culture, length (extensive rather than brief), and absence of fun and delight (Greaves 1992).

The *contamination and contagion hypothesis* holds that reports of ritualistic abuse are easily and unwittingly brought about when patients unconsciously incorporate the materials of others or do so for secondary gain. I return to this problem later in the chapter when I discuss the MPD (DID) subculture.

Greaves (1992) notes that some, finding other hypotheses lacking, have speculated an *extrasensory perception (ESP) hypothesis* and a *collective unconscious hypothesis,* holding that the material must come from somewhere, perhaps the unknown or the deep unconscious. He also cites Stanley Krippner's *personal myth hypothesis,* whereby the patient develops a personal allegory that expresses deep underlying truths in a way that he or she can attempt to live out. It is a personal rather than historical truth. The *propagation of rumor hypothesis* certainly has been demonstrated to be a powerful factor in generating public hysteria about satanism (e.g., Victor 1990). However, the individual accounts of patients usually do not have the characteristics of the rumors that lead to massive propagation among large populations. Most rumors that influence large groups of people do not involve specific first-person accounts related to and by specific people. Instead, they are secondhand or have a sufficient vagueness of attribution that they can take on a life of their own without being checked, confronted, and contradicted straightforwardly before gathering considerable momentum. Nonetheless, rumor may be a powerful factor among the MPD (DID) subculture.

Moving beyond the issues raised by Greaves (1992), it is useful to note that there is no reason to discount the possibility that some of the reports may be epiphenomena of psychotic illnesses. However, it is impressive to note that in a career of working with severely disturbed patients, I and the colleagues with whom I have discussed this issue have rarely if ever found structured accounts of satanic ritual abuse in schizophrenic or bipolar patients who did not have concomitant posttraumatic or dissociative psychopathology.

7. *Some patients are particularly vulnerable to misperceiving fantasy and/or illusion as reality and incorporate false beliefs into their autobiographical memory.* I will not address this theory in depth because it is explored elsewhere in this volume (see Barber, Chapter 2, and Bradford, Chapter 10), but I will note a few essential observations. Some individuals possess characteristics that render them more vulnerable than others to perceiving illusory experiences as compellingly as historical events and to accepting experiences of this nature into their autobiographical memories and personal constructs of reality. Spiegel (1974) and Spiegel and Spiegel (1978) described Grade 5 syndrome, and Wilson and Barber (1982) depicted the fantasy-prone personality, epitomizing this family of observations on illusion as reality. These studies are related to the general study of highly hypnotizable populations (see also Fraser, Chapter 6, in this volume).

Spiegel (1974) and Spiegel and Spiegel (1978) characterized the highly hypnotizable person with Grade 5 syndrome as having the following traits: a posture of trust in interpersonal situations, a ready and rapid suspension of critical judgment, an affiliation with new events, a relatively telescoped sense of time, an excellent memory, a fixed personality core, role confusion (due to both extreme malleability and hard-fixed dynamics), and sluggishness in reorienting to internal clues. Wilson and Barber (1982) found that many of their subjects believed their fantasies to be vivid and realistic experiences.

The patient with high dissociative capacity has a constellation of traits that overlaps with highly hypnotizable and fantasy-prone individuals. Ganaway (1989) observed that virtually all of the MPD (DID) patients under his observation qualified for Grade 5 syndrome, but this impressionistic statement was made without objective measures of hypnotizability and cannot be accepted as definitive. It is my impression that although many hospitalized MPD (DID) patients have these Grade 5 syndrome characteristics, many do not. Among highly functioning MPD (DID) outpatients, these characteristics are not as widely evident.

Clearly, most of the patients who allege ritualistic abuse have characteristics that force the circumspect clinician to consider that their vulnerabilities may have predisposed them to be influenced by many of the factors previously noted.

All of these hypotheses are not mutually exclusive. In a given patient, a number of factors may be at play. It is tempting to leap to the conclusion that one or more of them explain away the clinical phenomena in question, but this conclusion may prove more reassuring to the clinician than conducive to the patient's improvement. In my experience, it is usually wise to withhold premature conclusions in this complex and largely unresolved area.

Multiple Personality Disorder and Multiple Reality Disorder

Elsewhere (Kluft 1991, 1993a, 1993b), I have elaborated the observation that in patients with separate self-structures consistent with the clinical definitions of personalities and personality states—MPD (DID) patients and patients with dissociative disorder not otherwise specified (DDNOS) with the structure of MPD (DID)—the presence of alters with different worldviews, memory bands, and cognitive idiosyncrasies and errors results in the patient's endorsing mutually incompatible constructs of reality in the different alters. The resultant multiple reality disorder has the potential to render the patient intermittently psychotic with respect to consensually accepted constructs of reality.

Consequently, such a patient may represent his or her parents as ideal in one alter, as abusive in another, and as stalwarts of a satanic cult in another, and may deny they are his or her parents in another. It must not be assumed that the problematic distortions are invariably elaborations of abuse scenarios. I have seen many instances in which the patient held fast to a delusionally idealized image of an abusive parent who was incarcerated for incest and/or attempted murder of the patient or a sibling.

The crucial clinical fact is that many patients will be encountered who endorse alternative constructions of reality and who may be vulnerable to the induction of pseudomemories by the patients themselves, the unwary clinician, or other persons, pressures, or influences in their environment. In my clinical experiences, among the most vexing dilemmas is assessing the patient who alleges mistreatment, ritual or otherwise, but who has already spent months consulting with friends, coreligionists, fellow patients, and other clinicians and watching provocative talk shows before presenting at my office.

I recently was asked to assess the alleged ritualized abuse of a youngster in the context of a custody dispute. The girl's mother was a member of a religious group that believes that the devil and his minions walked the earth, which is a battleground between good and evil. She had been in treatment with a therapist who believed in ritual abuse and was supervised by a religiously oriented practitioner who claimed to be a survivor of ritual abuse. Encouraged by her therapist, she had repeatedly quizzed her daughter about ritual abuse experiences for months. After initial perplexity, the child began to endorse and elaborate ritual abuse experiences. Soon, she had implicated all paternal relatives and most immediate neighbors. The mother shared these data with her minister and congregation, who supported her in her battle to save her daughter and her daughter's soul.

My assessment of the girl revealed no stigmata of any abuse, but she clearly was being torn asunder by pressures generated by her warring parents. She had dissociated profoundly to accommodate their alternative views of reality.

In another custody dispute case, a young girl was being told by both parents that she was not being mistreated by them. Each parent painted for the child and the courts a portrait of blissful perfection in his or her relations with the girl while accusing the other of abusing her. The child was highly dissociated and had a diagnosable dissociative disorder. Although she denied any mistreatment at all, there was objective evidence of abuse, and the accounts of other parties allowed a reasonable determination of the guilty individual.

Tragically, despite energetic treatment for both of these youngsters, the illusory realities into which they had been indoctrinated remain more compelling than the actual realities suggested by incontrovertible evidence.

Interpersonal Ecology and Treating Patients Alleging Ritualistic Abuse: Notes on the Abuse Victim/ Multiple Personality Disorder Subculture

It is important to have a reasonably sophisticated appreciation of the forces that may affect the patient who alleges satanic or other forms of ritualized abuse. Previous discussions (e.g., Greaves 1992; Mulhern 1991) have focused on the therapist, the media, and society as sources of potential contamination. The impact of formal and informal networks of information exchange among patient populations—exchanges that create subcultures in which both information and disinformation can be disseminated with facility—also warrants consideration. Although these observations on information exchange might have been included earlier in this chapter, in the discussions of contagion and like phenomena, unique considerations are raised that merit a separate discussion.

Many MPD (DID)/DDNOS and other groups of patients, victims, and survivors are passionate students of the literature relating to their conditions; many express an intense desire, verbalized as an urgent need, to meet and network with fellow patients in the ostensible search for mutual support and validation. Friendships often spring up among these individuals, and support groups for victims or survivors of many varieties can be found in most cities and towns. Some are invaluable, and some are hothouses for promulgating psychopathology. I am particularly wary about leaderless or peer-facilitated support groups for dissociative disorder patients and others who allege that they are survivors of ritualistic abuse. I have tracked the course of more than a dozen of these groups over the years, and all but one were unmitigated disasters. As a rule, they began with great enthusiasm and high hopes, and, after their first months or year in the group, members reported that they were highly pleased with the group. However, all but one ended in retraumatizing significant fractions of their memberships. Recently, a colleague told me of a recovering MPD (DID) patient's reaction to attending a peer-facilitated support group for MPD (DID) patients: "A self-help group? No way! It was a self-helpless group!" This comment refers to the proclivity of these groups for overwhelming their members with one another's traumatic material, excessive dependency, and unbridled requests for support and nurture. It also refers to the possibility that members will, under the aegis of group forces and their own vulnerabilities, come to believe that they too have experienced what others represent as their personal histories. Furthermore, many of the group members have or form friendships with other group members so that exposing one to the issues of another can become a powerful force of which their therapists may remain more or less unaware.

Information networks are by no means limited to direct personal contacts. Several computer bulletin boards make it possible for individuals to contact one another worldwide, and many publications (with a spectrum of responsibility) address their concerns. The impact of this networking was underlined recently when a patient was discharged unexpectedly early from my own dissociative disorders program. Within half an hour, I had received several calls from patients asking if they could be admitted. I learned that a patient on our unit had called a friend about the opening, and that friend had put it on computer mail to those with whom she corresponded.

These subcultures and the information disseminated within and among them may be powerful determinants of what the therapist is told by a patient. That patient may, without any conscious intent to deceive self or therapist, bring into treatment materials that are not part of the patient's historical autobiographical experience but have become imbricated within the patient's autobiographical memory. I do not know to what extent these factors play a role in what is presented as clinical phenomenology and material. But I can share the personal observation that among those MPD (DID) patients and allegers of satanic ritual abuse whom I have treated, those who have networked extensively with fellow patients or allegers almost invariably take longer to treat than those who do not, and their treatment runs a stormier course. I currently refuse to treat patients who insist on participating in potentially contaminating and countertherapeutic activities. Their treatment is difficult enough without spending additional time and effort in dealing with the vicissitudes of subculture relationships and in trying to sort out which events may have been part of their experience and which may have been adopted from other sources.

Clinical Observations on Treating Patients Alleging Ritualistic Abuse

In this section, I address selected topics of clinical interest to practitioners working with patients who allege ritualistic abuse. I discuss several aspects of the dynamic significance of alleged ritualistic abuse.

The Ritualistic Abuse Account as Object-Coercive Diversion

Although many applaud the diminishing prominence of psychoanalytic thinking in contemporary psychotherapy training, I lament the forfeiture of generations of clinical wisdom that has accompanied this transition. For example, one of the basic questions the psychoanalytic practitioner asks is "Why is the patient bringing up this material at this moment in the therapy?" The psychodynamic and transferential implications of the structure of these choices are often profound. These implications are discussed in depth elsewhere (S. S. Marmer and R. P. Kluft, manuscript in preparation). Here, I explore one relevant aspect of this psychoanalytic perspective, object-coercive diversion, and comment on several themes with clear psychoanalytic dimensions under a number of other headings as well. The contemporary psychoanalytically oriented clinician may consult Gabbard (1994) for a useful overview.

Kramer (1983) described the defense of object-coercive doubting in response to maternal incest. The young women Kramer studied had mothers who had perceived their daughters as imperfect, had devalued and abused them, and had not allowed them to individuate. Torn by their split perceptions of their mothers, her young female subjects "coerced the maternal object or her substitute to argue one of the opposing sides of the child's intrapsychic conflict (or its derivative)"(p. 331). In arguments that usually related to polarized perceptions of an object, or whether something was known or not or had occurred or not, there was "almost never any closure to the conflict" (p. 332).

The similarity between the coercive pressures exerted by Kramer's young patients and the behavior of dissociative patients, especially those alleging ritualized abuse, has long impressed me. Often, dissociative patients will exert strong and sustained pressure on me to either validate or repudiate the alleged ritualistic abuse experiences, as if to externalize one pole of his or her uncertainty and make me its champion, at which point the patient may take the other point of view either at once or in the future. This behavior may be termed an *object-coercive diversion.*

Object-coercive diversion allows the therapy to become decentered from coping with here-and-now realities, transference, and significant object relations. Instead, the sessions are subverted into a series of quests to attain the unreachable goal of certainty as to whether the ritualized abuse is or was real, and attaining the unreachable goal is established as a precondition of recovery, which therefore cannot be achieved. I will be reproached for failing to validate my patient's personal truth, thereby creating a critical, distrustful, and uncaring atmosphere that precludes the sense of safety and acceptance that is a precondition for my patient's recovery. Or, I will be chastised for persuading [sic] my patient that some preposterous and impossible event or events have occurred and causing an irretrievable breach between my patient and those he or she loves and needs in his or her life in order to be well. Under such conditions, an interminable or stalemated treatment becomes inevitable. It is essential to become sensitized to the fact that although accounts of ritualistic abuse may prove to be derivatives of crucial issues, they may be presented as object-coercive diversion. Object-coercive diversions should not be joined; they should receive what Chu (1992) has described as "compassionate confrontation" and tactful interpretation.

Although many therapists genuinely believe the axiom that a good therapist must believe his or her patient, in my opinion and experience this is a completely wrongheaded notion that verges on the foolish and fatuous. Instead, I would submit that the message coming through in studying the psychoanalysis literature is that the good therapist must believe in his or her patient and what the patient may become with the help of treatment. Even during the treatment of a neurotic patient, he or she will offer many different perspectives on a given event or relationship in the course of its exploration.

It becomes important to appreciate, as best one can, why and how a preoccupation with coercing the therapist into the role of arbiter of historical reality has assumed prominence. The conflict over what is real or not to the patient is a conflict of the patient's. When this conflict becomes the preoccupation of the therapist, through externalization, projection, projective identification, introjective identification, or entrapment in object-coercive doubting (which combines many of these mechanisms), something is very wrong. The forte of the therapist is care and healing, not detective work. All too often, when external evidence confirms things one way or another, the patient remains unchanged. We serve the patient best when we work toward the patient's recovery. The patient who attributes magical properties to hypnosis, drug-facilitated interviews, or the therapist's perspicacity has to be helped, gently and compassionately, to hold a more moderate view of what is possible.

The patient's wish to be confirmed in his or her beliefs often is an outgrowth of the patient's sense of unlovability and rejectability. He or she feels unworthy and ashamed, ruined, and beyond help. The patient cannot believe he or she is accepted by the therapist and searches for a way to prove he or she deserves or is entitled to the therapist's care and concern. Often, one's quest to be believed is undertaken to demonstrate that one's pain and need are real and compel attention. Just as often, the patient may reenact a childhood attempt to get others to perceive the child's pain and rescue the child. Unfortunately, what is being reenacted is almost inevitably the experience of being disbelieved and repudiated as a child. The therapist will be tested repeatedly and pressed into the position of either confirming the patient's account or being considered dangerous or untrustworthy.

The integrity of both the therapist and the therapy is best served by defining the reality of what is revealed as a problem to be addressed in therapy rather than by attempting to solve it apodictically or auctorially.

Why It May Be Desirable to Recall Having Experienced Ritualistic Abuse

The potential for object-coercive diversion by a patient reporting ritualized abuse is impressive, especially in psychotherapy conducted by a therapist who either is unfamiliar with managing reports of ritualized abuse or takes the stance that such accounts are, as a rule, completely factual or completely false. The painful process of integrating one's psyche and changing one's maladaptive patterns and pursuits may be brought to an effective halt; in fact, the psychopathology may be sanctioned as a reasonable pattern of response to genuine external threat. The resistance is effectively reinforced by the therapist.

Furthermore, working through problematic relationships, facing essential reality concerns, and wrestling with crucial decisions may be deferred as the patient remains preoccupied with horrendous events that may not have occurred and cult-related abusers who may not have existed or who may be the screens on which are projected convoluted fantasies misperceived as realities. Not uncommonly, the patient remains enmeshed with and unable to work on issues related to an abusive family while remaining totally dysfunctional and preoccupied with the ceremonies and routines alleged to be associated with a ritual calendar. The displacement of concerns onto a mysterious cult leaves more important, albeit more commonplace, concerns unattended. In another variant, all relationships with a family of origin may be severed, and the patient may live in fear of the family and the cult making efforts to reinvolve him or her.

Being preoccupied with and experiencing anguish about the cult, however terrible, may be more tolerable for the patient than the prospect of acknowledging that significant others have betrayed and exploited the patient for no reason more exalted than their self-indulgence, depravity, or mental abnormality. A focus on cultic concerns forestalls for many the pain of grieving for the idealizations and residual longings for connectedness with important objects to whom they retain affectionate, albeit conflictual, attachments. Grief, despair, and the end of hope that things could be otherwise are effectively deferred.

Introducing charges of cultic involvement may be helpful to arrest the interest of the therapist, to fascinate and inspire pity in the therapist for the survivor of such horrors, to intimidate the therapist (e.g., "They know I am seeing you, and they said that they are watching you!"), or to divert the treatment from anxiety-provoking areas. It may be difficult to appreciate that the apparent horror demonstrated by patients may be more tolerable than the issues from which cultic concerns deflect treatment. Many patients find it easier to recount endless tales of ritualized atrocities than to assert themselves with their families or to work toward returning to employment. Accounts of participating in a transgenerational cult may be used by patients to aggrandize their own importance, to suggest that their mistreatment had a larger purpose, or to demonstrate that their ambivalently perceived family members are not simply abusive and responsible for their actions, but are themselves participants in an ongoing tradition into which they were similarly initiated. Perversely, these accounts allow patients to retain hope that they will someday be reconciled with their families.

Other possible benefits to alleging a history of ritualistic abuse may be a reaction formation to one's own aggression and sadistic fantasies; a particularly potent (and narcissistically invested) expression of one's masochism; a plea for sympathy and exoneration from responsibility; an effort to legitimize one's voracious dependency needs and prolonged disability; an expression of being special and unique; a form of exhibitionistic, narcissistic, and grandiose self-presentation; and a method of defeating the potency of the therapy and the therapist.

C. G. Fine (personal communications, August 1993–March 1994) has described MPD (DID) patients who use ritualized abuse accounts as a conscious screen. Fine's description is related to Kluft's (1993a, 1993b) characterization of MPD (DID) as multiple reality disorder. From Kluft's perspective, some alters are convinced of alternative constructions of reality (e.g., ritualized abuse). Others consciously know that this is not the case but do not contradict the former's beliefs because the deception serves other adaptational and intrapsychic purposes.

This discussion of why patients recall ritualistic abuse experiences is fragmentary and incomplete and does not repeat other possible mechanisms mentioned throughout this chapter. However, it may serve to underline the complexities that must be considered when we study the question, Why would anyone want to lie about something so horrible? The implicit trailer or conclusion to this question is, It must be true. Such simplicity of thinking discards much of what we have learned about psychodynamics.

This statement, however, in no way contradicts the possibility of the genuine existence of ritualized abuse and leaves open the possibility that all of the mechanisms proposed in this chapter might be co-opted by those who wish to discount the existence of ritualistic abuse to discredit that possibility. My own practice is strongly influenced by my former mentor and his core conflictual relationship theme (CCRT) methodology (Luborsky 1984). I use his methodology, illustrated in the following clinical vignettes:

Case 1

Recently, I oversaw the treatment of several young women who alleged horrendous experiences in satanic cults and maintained that the cult was still after them. The first was a highly exhibitionistic young woman, unwilling to focus on major issues, who was attention seeking at every opportunity. Verbatim notes of her self-expression revealed a consistent CCRT, in all contexts, related to her wish to be admired and attended to. When satanic accounts did not lead to her receiving the attention she craved, she began to talk about her ties to the Mafia. Although she claimed the cult and the Mafia were still after her, she suffered no untoward consequences and found employment and gratification as an exotic dancer. I tentatively concluded that the cultic allegations were unlikely and the material was reported in the service of her idiosyncratic dynamics.

Case 2

A second patient alleging ritualized abuse had MPD (DID) and recurrent major depression with psychotic features. Following her CCRTs, I determined that cultic material emerged in strength only in the context of episodes of psychotic depression and then was recalled but neither embroidered further nor a part of her recurrent CCRTs when her affective disorder was under control. I determined that the cultic abuse ideas were an expression of her negativistic delusions while affectively psychotic. Kept on maintenance antidepressants and treated for MPD (DID), she has recovered and rarely alludes to the cultic material, which she increasingly understands to be delusional material unwittingly incorporated into her autobiographical memory.

Case 3

A third patient had nearly integrated her MPD (DID) when a life crisis caused her to be hospitalized on a dissociative disorders unit where ritualistic abuse was widely discussed. She became concerned that she might have suffered ritualistic abuse. On discharge, she reported memories of ritualistic abuse for the first time. In regular or hypnotic sessions, there was no other material or CCRT theme to support these memories. I decided to work on the hypothesis that these memories were due to contamination, but I explored them with her as any other material in treatment. The memories of ritual abuse rapidly ceased and did not recur in the subsequent 5 years. She has been integrated and fully employed for 4 years.

Case 4

A fourth patient with MPD (DID) never talked to others about her memories of ritualistic abuse. Her intrafamilial abuse is well documented in legal records. Much of it is admitted by her mother, who was a prostitute, and some was witnessed by her sister, whose abuse is also well documented. She worked through ritual abuse memories and recovered. Her CCRTs have been consistent throughout treatment. Another patient has given accounts that buttress this patient's allegations in great detail. In the treatment, the material on ritualistic abuse was addressed as if it had both historical and psychological reality. Information on ritualistic abuse made available by the patient and others does not suggest or allow the peremptory discounting of her reports of being a victim of ritualized abuse, nor does it allow matter-of-fact acceptance as true in whole or in part.

Case 5

A fifth patient was found to have a pattern of introducing material on ritualistic abuse to arrest her therapist's attention whenever she felt that her therapist was drawing away from her. Nonetheless, at all times her CCRTs suggested a view of the world permeated by anticipating horrible mistreatment. On many occasions throughout her therapy, her allegations appeared to be either consistent or inconsistent, only to have the balance shift once again. In the face of this confusing welter of impressions, the patient and therapist were able to focus on the patient's here-and-now adaptation and peacefulness among her system of alters, an approach that led to slow but gratifying improvement.

Must Memories of Ritualistic Abuse Be Addressed in Treatment?

It would be useful to determine whether allegations of ritualized abuse must be addressed or could be bypassed with impunity. Although many prominent clinicians have offered contradictory opinions on this matter, their observations and advice must be contextualized and considered with some skepticism to appreciate the implications of their recommendations. Clinicians do not treat uniform populations. Those who are highly skeptical about the reality of alleged ritualistic abuse often hear that patients making these allegations rapidly abandon them. Minimizing the allegations is advocated. Those who are more open to the possibility of ritualistic abuse often hear that extensive abreactive work is useful in relieving these patients and is essential to their recovery. Cautious, systematic exploration and abreaction of allegations are advocated.

However, in practice, patients and their families or loved ones often opt for a treatment program that has one orientation or the other. Their expectations and implied values and priorities are congenial with the philosophy of the treatment program they enter, and compliance with the proposed regimen follows naturally. In my own program, we have steadfastly refused to endorse either polar view. Patients who inquire about our philosophy on allegations of ritualistic abuse usually are disappointed, and those searching for a congenial polarized view rarely decide to enter our program.

In my experience, no firm generalizations can be offered. Some of the following information in this chapter is derived from my clinical work and is refined anecdotal information at best. It is always best, whenever possible, to defer work on traumatic material until the patient is thoroughly assessed, is confident in the commitment of the therapist to the patient and the therapy, has been strengthened, and has become able, with the help of the therapist, to contain difficult material so that it does not overwhelm the patient between sessions (Fine 1991; Kluft 1993a, 1993b).

During these early stages of treatment, which are discussed in another context later in this chapter, the therapist and patient can begin to explore what role the allegations of ritual abuse play in the overall psychopathology of the patient and what factors may contribute to the patient's making such reports. Evidence suggesting actual involvement and alternative hypotheses for the origins of the allegations can be acquired while getting to know the patient. It also may prove possible to ascertain the psychodynamic contexts in which the patient begins to raise ritualized abuse material. Luborsky's (1984) CCRT methodology has often served me well in this connection. In one particularly thorny situation in which urgent action based on my best understanding was necessary, I was able to reconstruct from my verbatim notes that every time the patient began to fear rejection by me or my colleague, she introduced material suggesting we were the objects of cult assassination plans and that only assiduous attention to her every utterance might yield the information necessary to protect ourselves. I gradually made interpretations with this understanding in mind, and the cultic material and threats faded into the background as we explored her desperate wish to be loved and her profound separation issues.

Therapy begins with the exploration of more mundane experiences. At this point, one of several patterns usually asserts itself. In the first pattern, the patient becomes deeply involved in treatment and digs in. The ritualistic material is heard with decreasing frequency, and the patient gradually recovers without its achieving prominence and requiring significant work. The inference is drawn that this ritualistic material was an allegory for the actual material, although the alternative hypothesis that actual ritual abuse experiences were worked out through derivative productions has not been disproved.

In the second pattern, after a phase of working through more mundane material, the ritualistic material surfaces and demands attention. The patient improves as the material is worked through. The inference may be drawn that the ritualistic material was more upsetting and therefore more deeply repressed or dissociated or that the patient is not yet ready to leave the therapist and is generating more sensational material to prolong the therapist's interest and investment in the patient.

A third pattern is that the material on ritualistic abuse assumes prominence early in the therapy and cannot be put aside. Efforts to do so collapse repeatedly. The inference may be drawn that the pain of this material is so intense that the need to address it is overwhelming, or that the patient is still active in ritualistic abuse situations, or that the metaphorical or allegorical expression of more mundane experiences and conflicts through ritualistic abuse material is essential in the patient's psychological economy and serves a displacement or a screen function. There is no alternative to working through the material as it is presented because its psychological reality to the patient is intense and compelling, and the symptomatic behaviors alleged to have their origins in experiences of ritualistic abuse dominate the clinical landscape. Treatment usually runs a prolonged course, and patients often have a guarded prognosis.

If the material on ritualistic abuse continues to be accorded a profoundly important psychological reality by the patient, it will have to be addressed despite uncertainty about its historical reality. The skeptical but compassionate clinician may take some reassurance and consolation from the frequent observation that since the time of the first shamans, patients have been getting well through treatments that were accepted by both healer and patient but were not based on scientifically accepted principles and established truths (Ellenberger 1970). Many patients are being treated successfully in past-lives therapies that, according to current scientific beliefs, lack a credible empirical foundation.

What Is the Bottom-Line Effect of a Patient's Alleging Ritualistic Abuse?

Unpublished data accumulated in the course of developing an instrument to measure treatment progress strongly suggest that an MPD (DID) patient's allegation of ritualistic abuse is associated with a near doubling of the length of treatment (Kluft 1994) and a higher likelihood of crises, regressions, hospitalizations, and episodes of self-injury. It is not clear whether these findings are due to the severity of traumatization inflicted under circumstances of ritualistic abuse, complication of the treatment by exogenous factors associated with alternative hypotheses about the etiology and perpetuation of accounts of ritualistic abuse, or complication of the treatment by endogenous factors in patients who can be induced or can induce themselves, deliberately or unwittingly, to allege ritualized abuse.

Principles for Treating Patients Alleging Ritualistic Abuse

The following principles have served me well in working with patients who make allegations in therapy that can neither be proved nor disproved and whose therapies make active efforts to explore their pasts, efforts that in and of themselves may alter their perceptions of their personal histories. These principles are derived primarily from work with patients who allege incest and/or ritualistic abuse experiences.

Explain the Principle of Informed Uncertainty

When the patient and I are embarking on a voyage together over the stormy and uncharted seas of the patient's memory, and what will be discovered may have a powerful impact on the treatment and the patient's life, I try to offer the patient a realistic perspective on future possibilities of uncertainty in understanding material elicited in therapy. I follow Appelbaum and Gutheil (1982, 1991; numerous lectures by and personal communications with T. G. Gutheil over many years) in offering the patient a realistic perspective as an aspect of informed consent:

> Informed consent, appropriately conceptualized, represents an atmosphere of openness and honesty, nurtured by an ongoing dialogue between clinician and patient that begins from the first encounter and lasts for the duration of the relationship. It is not a brief conversation, capped by the patient's signature on a form, which renders the issue closed. The model . . . has been described as a "process model" of informed consent . . . where differing perceptions of illness, values, and expectations are shared in a manner termed "mutual monitoring" by patient and clinician. (Appelbaum and Gutheil 1991, p. 183)

In this model, the therapist empathizes with the patient's unrealistic wishes in a manner that brings them into the open and allows gradual disillusionment of the patient from those magical wishes and fantasies. For example, the following verbalizations are closely modeled on those of Appelbaum and Gutheil (1991, pp. 183–184):

> I wish that the good Lord had provided us with a method to distinguish accurate memories from inaccurate ones, but unfortunately that has not yet been granted to us. Therefore, it is important not to rush to conclusions or to take hasty actions on the basis of what appear to be memories. We will need to explore them in depth and at length.

I wish I could assure you that I could judge from your genuine anguish and the horrible things you have described with complete conviction that these things had occurred in the very way that you described. Unhappily, we just cannot be sure about these things—our science has not advanced that far.

I wish I could assure you that what comes up under hypnosis (or in Amytal interviews or in your nightmares) represents what has happened to you in the past. Unfortunately, we do not know how to be sure in such circumstances, and all we can be reasonably confident of is that what we find may be useful in suggesting hypotheses for further exploration.

I try to elicit my patient's expectations and beliefs about memory, treatment, and any specific techniques (such as hypnosis) that may be employed. I make efforts to correct any erroneous impressions. I make detailed inquiry to confirm that my planned interventions will not have a deleterious impact on my patient's other priorities. For example, I will not employ hypnosis if it seems likely that the patient might later become a litigant, defendant, or witness in court, where his or her having been hypnotized may be understood to have undermined the credibility of his or her memory.

I review with the patient what is known about the subjects at hand and share what is often said by polarized experts and media pundits. It is difficult indeed if a treatment gets under way without this step, given the vicissitudes of the media and vagaries of talk-show sensationalism.

I review the implications of those steps for the treatment process and anticipate particular difficulties unique to the patient's situation. I explain in depth and at length that recovery does not necessarily require discovering the absolute truth and attempt to deal with the patient's shock at this revelation. I indicate that honesty and the truth are important but take pains to indicate that there are severe limitations on their determination. I outline the potential benefits and liabilities of the treatment and the techniques discussed.

I explain that the problems with which we will be forced to contend do not reside exclusively in the past, the therapist, the patient, or the therapy and that problematic influences may occur outside of treatment as well as within it. This communicated, I ask the patient to verbalize his or her understanding of what I have said and correct any misperceptions. I insist that the new understanding be verbalized and corrected again if need be.

Only then do I document that informed consent can be given and that it has been given. In selected cases, I may do this in writing. In unusual and infrequent situations, I may insist that the entire therapy be recorded as a safeguard.

Consider Informed Consent as a Continuing Process

Because of the nature of psychotherapy, especially with dissociative patients and those alleging ritualized abuse, it is essential that therapists be aware that issues addressed with these patients need to be readdressed repeatedly. Magical expectations die hard, if at all. The therapist contending with multiple reality disorder in MPD (DID) or any other highly dissociation-prone individual may suddenly come to appreciate that there is little carryover of his or her efforts from one discrete state of consciousness with its associated construction of reality and another. Rarely a month passes in treating a patient alleging ritualized abuse without the need to reexplore such concerns. In workshop settings, I often remark that "hope springs infernal" to convey how persistently the patient's request for magical reassurances springs to life again and again.

Remember, the Perfect Is the Enemy of the Good

It is often tempting to submit to the rigors of an unrealistic therapeutic or investigational superego or to aspire to match an impossible ego ideal. We would like to believe that we can discover the truth about our patients and submit reluctantly, if at all, to acknowledging the extent of our confusions and uncertainties. This uncertainty is not alleviated by the patient's recurrent efforts to put us in the position of arbiter of what is true or not true. We serve our patients, if not our vanities, best if we keep the limitations of our knowledge and abilities to discern the truth firmly in the forefront of our considerations. Overestimating our abilities is at best a narcissistic defense and at worst hubris, leading inevitably to our decline and fall, the victims of our tragic flaws. The welfare of our patients is linked to our honesty and integrity and will plummet as well, and this is intolerable. We are at risk of discarding the Hippocratic injunction—"First, do no harm"—if we enter into a parallel process and collude with our patients' dysfunctional wishes that we see ourselves as so transcendently wise that we are entitled to create from unreliable data and endorse a construct of reality that may prove to be inaccurate and tainted by our unacknowledged grandiosity.

Never Forsake the Role of Healer and the Practice of Healing Arts

When dealing with the patient who alleges ritualistic abuse, we can heal far more than we can understand. Most therapists are terrible detectives and lack grounding in the rudiments of criminal investigation, sociology, anthropology, and many other relevant areas of expertise. Withdrawal into the stance of the dispassionate investigator is inconsistent with the intense and intimate involvement that characterizes successful therapy. Conan Doyle's famous detective Sherlock Holmes worked within a model that allowed him to observe, with a charming arrogance, "It is a capital offense, Watson, to hypothesize in advance of the facts." We clinicians lack the luxury of Holmes's dispassion and objectivity. We are more the colleagues of Dr. Watson, condemned to exercise our bumbling and limited art, knowledge, and skills when our patients are in pain before us, all too often mortifyingly aware of the limitations of our knowledge. We must hypothesize, in the presence of human suffering, the type of fact to which our profession's knowledge, however imperfect, is dedicated, and often in advance of the facts that would establish the etiology of that suffering.

When I reflect on my work in my study at home, I am often disgruntled and upset that I have helped someone recover and return to healthy function without any real certainty about whether what we worked through in the treatment had actually occurred. However, when I am grappling with the patient's pain and psychopathology in my office, I am encouraged and gratified that despite its limitations, psychotherapy can alleviate as much despair and provide an anodyne to as much human pain and suffering as it can.

The patient alleging ritualistic abuse poses an enormous clinical challenge. We can meet that challenge best by marshaling the cumulative wisdom of psychotherapeutic practice and relevant scientific findings and bringing them to bear with compassion and circumspection in these unusual and trying circumstances.

In my study is a statue of an Inuit shaman transforming himself into the forms and spirits of various animals—the seal, the raven, the polar bear, and the beaver—to gain access to their special strengths and knowledge in order to understand and heal the afflicted. At my desk, I search among my books on psychoanalysis, hypnosis, cognitive therapy, psychopharmacology, and other assorted approaches to appreciating and alleviating human discomfort. I wink at him as I write this—we are colleagues and brothers.

References

American Psychiatric Association: Diagnostic and Statistical Manual of Mental Disorders, 4th Edition. Washington, DC, American Psychiatric Association, 1994

Appelbaum PS, Gutheil TG: Clinical Handbook of Psychiatry and the Law. Baltimore, MD, Williams & Wilkins, 1982

Appelbaum PS, Gutheil TG: Clinical Handbook of Psychiatry and the Law, Second Edition. Baltimore, MD, Williams & Wilkins, 1991

Chu JA: Empathic confrontation in the treatment of childhood abuse survivors, including a tribute to the legacy of Dr. David Caul. Dissociation 5:98–103, 1992

Ellenberger HF: The Discovery of the Unconscious. New York, Basic Books, 1970

Fine CG: Treatment stabilization and crisis prevention: pacing the therapy of the MPD patient. Psychiatr Clin North Am 14:661–675, 1991

Friesen JG: Uncovering the Mystery of MPD. San Bernardino, CA, Here's Life Publishers, 1991

Gabbard GO: Psychodynamic Psychiatry in Clinical Practice: The DSM-IV Edition. Washington, DC, American Psychiatric Press, 1994

Ganaway GK: Historical truth versus narrative truth: clarifying the role of exogenous trauma in the etiology of multiple personality disorder and its variants. Dissociation 2:205–220, 1989

Ganaway GK: Satanic ritual abuse: critical issues and alternative hypotheses. Panel presentation at the Seventh International Conference on Multiple Personality Disorder/Dissociative States, Chicago, IL, November 1990

Goodwin J: Munchausen's syndrome as a dissociative disorder. Dissociation 1:54–60, 1988

Greaves GB: Alternative hypotheses regarding claims of satanic cult activity: a critical analysis, in Out of Darkness: Exploring Satanism and Ritual Abuse. Edited by Sakheim DK, Devine SE. New York, Lexington Books, 1992, pp 45–72

Hill S, Goodwin J: Satanism: similarities between patient accounts and pre-Inquisition historical sources. Dissociation 2:39–44, 1989

Kluft RP: Treatment of multiple personality disorder. Psychiatr Clin North Am 7:9–29, 1984

Kluft RP: The parental fitness of mothers with multiple personality disorder: a preliminary study. Child Abuse Negl 11:273–280, 1987

Kluft RP: Multiple personality disorder, in American Psychiatric Press Review of Psychiatry, Vol 10. Edited by Tasman A, Goldfinger SM. Washington, DC, American Psychiatric Press, 1991, pp 161–188

Kluft RP: The initial stages of psychotherapy in the treatment of multiple personality disorder patients. Dissociation 6:145–161, 1993a

Kluft RP: The treatment of dissociative disorder patients: an overview of discoveries, successes, and failures. Dissociation 6:87–101, 1993b

Kluft RP: Treatment trajectories in multiple personality disorder. Dissociation 7:63–74, 1994

Kramer S: Object-coercive doubting: a pathological response to maternal incest. J Am Psychoanal Assoc 31 (suppl):325–351, 1983

Lanning KV: Ritual abuse: a law enforcement perspective. Child Abuse Negl 15:171–173, 1991

Luborsky L: Principles of Psychoanalytic Psychotherapy. New York, Basic Books, 1984

Mulhern S: Satanism and psychotherapy: a rumor in search of an inquisition, in The Satanism Scare. Edited by Richardson JT, Best J, Bromley DG. New York, Aldine De Gruyter, 1991, pp 145–172

Noll R: Vampires, Werewolves, and Demons: Twentieth Century Case Reports in the Psychiatric Literature. New York, Brunner/Mazel, 1992

Putnam FW: The satanic ritual abuse controversy. Child Abuse Negl 15:175–179, 1991

Ross CA: Satanic Ritual Abuse: Principles of Treatment. Toronto, Ontario, University of Toronto Press, 1995

Smith M, Pazder L: Michelle Remembers. New York, Pocket Books, 1980

Spiegel H: The Grade 5 syndrome: the highly hypnotizable person. Int J Clin Exp Hypn 22:303–319, 1974

Spiegel H, Spiegel D: Trance and Treatment: Clinical Uses of Hypnosis. New York, Basic Books, 1978

Van Benschoten SC: Multiple personality disorders and satanic ritual abuse: the issue of credibility. Dissociation 3:22–30, 1990

Victor JS: The spread of satanic cult rumors. Skeptical Inquirer 14:287–291, 1990

Wilson SC, Barber TX: The fantasy-prone personality: implications for understanding imagery, hypnosis and parapsychological phenomena, in Imagery: Current Theory, Research, and Application. Edited by Sheikh A. New York, Wiley, 1982, pp 340–387

Young WC, Sachs RG, Braun BG, et al: Patients reporting ritual abuse in childhood: a clinical syndrome: report of 37 cases. Child Abuse Negl 15:181–189, 1991

Recognition and Special Treatment Issues in Patients Reporting Childhood Sadistic Ritual Abuse

Walter C. Young, M.D., F.A.P.A.
Linda J. Young, R.N.C., M.A.

*L*ess than a decade ago, sadistic ritual abuse (SRA) was considered an isolated and bizarre phenomenon. Young et al. (1991) described a syndrome of ritual abuse, including abuses reported by 37 patients (Table 4–1) and psychiatric sequelae for the patient population (Table 4–2). Today, increasing numbers of patients in the United States are reporting a history of childhood ritual abuse perpetrated by cults. These cults are described as transgenerational, geographically dispersed, networked, and often satanic (Gould 1987, 1992; Kelly 1988, 1989; Kinscherff and Barnum 1992; Sakheim and Devine 1992; Snow 1990; Young 1992; Young et al. 1991). Allegations of ritual abuse also have been reported in England (Jones 1991), the Netherlands (Jonker and Jonker-Bakker 1991), and Canada (Fraser 1990).

Descriptions of SRA have been met with a spectrum of reactions. At one end are therapists who accept all accounts as valid. At the other end are those who believe none of the reports are valid but instead reflect a social hysteria, a suggested syndrome passed

We acknowledge Kathleen Adams, M.A., for her editorial expertise.

Table 4–1.   Common abuses reported in sadistic ritual abuse cases

Sexual abuse
Witnessing and receiving physical abuse or torture
Witnessing animal mutilations or killings
Death threats
Forced drug use
Witnessing and forced participation in human adult and infant sacrifice
Forced cannibalism
Marriage to Satan
Buried alive in coffins or graves
Forced impregnation and sacrifice of own child

Source.   Adapted from Young et al. 1991.

Table 4–2.   Common psychiatric sequelae reported in sadistic ritual
abuse cases

Severe posttraumatic stress disorders[a]
Dissociative states with satanic overtones
Survivor guilt
Indoctrinated beliefs
Unusual fears
Sexualization of sadistic impulse
Bizarre self-abuse
Substance abuse

[a]Met criteria for DSM-III-R (American Psychiatric Association 1987).
Source.   Adapted from Young et al. 1991.

to patients by their therapists, or an elaborate metaphor for more
prosaic forms of childhood trauma (Ganaway 1989, 1990; Gardner
1992; Lanning 1991, 1992; Loftus and Ketcham 1994; Mulhern 1990,
1991; Noll 1989, 1990; Ofshe and Watters 1994; Putnam 1990, 1991;
Richardson et al. 1991; Victor 1993). A more moderate point of view
remains open-minded to these reports until data supporting a de-
fensible position are forthcoming (Greaves 1992; Hill and Goodwin
1989; Kluft 1989; Sakheim and Devine 1992; Van Benschoten 1990;
Young 1992; Young et al. 1991).

Although children also have reported incidents of ritual abuse
(Gould 1987, 1992; Kelly 1988, 1989; Kinscherff and Barnum 1992;
Snow 1990; Tennant-Clark et al. 1989), this chapter is limited to the

treatment of adults who report being abused as children. The population of patients reporting ritual abuse has changed during the past 10 years, even as this population is studied. For that reason, solid data have not been immediately available.

Certain problems confound our understanding of ritual abuse. For example, increasing numbers of people are suddenly reporting histories of ritual abuse, often with dramatic presentations, leading us to believe that a large portion of patients purported to be survivors are in fact merely camp followers, who for one reason or another malinger, unconsciously recall reports from elsewhere, or resurrect fantasies and assimilate them.

In addition, we are aware of many accounts of ritual abuse that were believed in absolutely and convincingly by patients but were simply found to be untrue. For these reasons, we have to understand that treatment and diagnostic considerations are tentative, and in some ways experimental, and subject to continuing evolution.

Perspectives from sociology and anthropology reveal a great deal about the propagation of mass psychogenic illnesses and rumor panics that appear to apply to the mushrooming spread of current ritual abuse reports. We must remain cautious not only in diagnosing and understanding these conditions, but also in understanding all issues surrounding memory and recall. Not that memory and recall may be inaccurate, but there is too much that we cannot yet substantiate to draw firm conclusions. However, we have yet to account for the significant psychopathy in these patients, which is not necessarily a feature seen in those individuals caught up in rumor panics of other varieties.

We propose in this chapter that treatment be based on the assumption that the patients' past experiences dictate the context and meaning of their symptoms and that their belief in this history is the basis of their behavior and emotional responses. It is the patients' presentation of behavior and emotional responses that dictates the course of their therapy. However, patients may receive a course of treatment for a condition based only on internal belief rather than historical accuracy. Nonetheless, there is a need to resolve their internal perceived conflict, which must not be ignored by the therapeutic community. The term *memory* is used to depict individuals' belief in what has occurred and does not imply historical accuracy.

Finally, treating patients in accordance with the material they present and in the context of their own belief systems is at present the best treatment we know. In the long term, other treatment techniques that are equally successful and lead to less painful outcomes may clarify cases where ritual abuse has not occurred and others where ritual abuse might have historical accuracy in some context.

Definition

The meaning of SRA in this chapter is limited to adults reporting childhood abuse, including "sadistic group torture and abuse of children . . . reported as intra-familial, transgenerational groups that engage in explicit satanic worship which includes reports of practices such as ritual torture, sacrificial murder, deviant sexual activity, and ceremonial cannibalism" (Young et al. 1991, p. 182). SRA is supposedly designed to gain control of the behaviors and beliefs of children and to obtain conformity to a set of quasi-religious teachings.

Purpose

The purpose of this chapter is to review reports of the SRA phenomenon, to discuss credibility of the accounts, and to describe current issues in its treatment, including preparation for treatment, general treatment issues, management of cultic or satanic alters, indoctrination issues, histories suggesting deceptive practices, pharmacological treatment, and controversy over historical accuracy. Controversial trends in the etiology and treatment of SRA cases are also discussed.

It should be kept in mind that the controversy surrounding SRA continues to heighten. Actual clinical interpretations may be considerably different if scientific data should support patients' accounts or, from an opposing viewpoint, if a socially contagious, media-influenced syndrome is shown to run its course among dissociative, suggestible individuals.

Recognition of Sadistic Ritual Abuse

Although SRA is not a formal diagnostic category, the terms *diagnostic* and *recognition* are used interchangeably in this chapter. Because patients with SRA recollection require specialized treatment strategies, the concept of its diagnosis as a recognized entity allows for the development of a specific treatment approach.

The relation between severe and prolonged childhood physical and sexual abuse and pronounced dissociation is well established (Braun 1986; Putnam 1985, 1989; Spiegel 1984, 1988). The dissociation may evolve along a spectrum of severity, with multiple personality disorder (MPD), more recently called dissociative identity disorder (DID) in DSM-IV (American Psychiatric Association 1994), being among the most disturbing of a variety of dissociative patterns. Contributing factors include age at onset of abuse, duration and severity of abuse, and constitutional and environmental factors.

SRA reportedly involves massive abuse, resulting in clinical symptoms that may lead to early recognition. These clinical symptoms include dissociative symptoms, posttraumatic stress disorder (PTSD) symptoms, cult-related phenomena, bizarre self-abuse, and unremitting eating, sleep, and anxiety disorders (see Table 4–2).

Dissociative Symptoms

Many patients reporting SRA present with severe dissociative symptoms, including MPD/DID. Therefore, a diagnosis of dissociation of MPD/DID remains the highest common factor in those reporting SRA. However, the converse, that all dissociative symptoms reflect SRA, does not logically follow.

Posttraumatic Stress Disorder Symptoms

Severe traumatic abuses (see Table 4–1) frequently lead to acute and chronic PTSD characterized by states of hyperarousal and autonomic nervous system lability alternating with periods of emotional constriction and withdrawal. There may be flashbacks with vivid sensory and kinesthetic images of trauma or repetitive nightmares relating to the trauma. PTSD may be present even though the patient has no apparent awareness of the source of trauma.

Cult-Related Phenomena

Flashbacks or memories of cultlike phenomena may emerge and dominate the PTSD syndrome. The patient may draw, write, dream, or talk about ceremonies or rituals, including descriptions of knives, blood, altars, robes, circles, animals, satanic symbols, and other cultlike experiences such as those shown in Table 4–1. When patients begin to describe these experiences, they may be flooded with scenes of group victimization in which multiple adults participate in or force the patient to witness the abuse of others.

Other early clinical signs suggesting SRA may come through the emergence of satanic or cultic alters, who generally present as hostile, destructive, aligned with satanic beliefs, and focused on the patient's punishment. These alters appear as identifications with so-called perpetrators and may present with a variety of cultlike names and functions.

Bizarre Self-Abuse

Frequent self-mutilation by cutting, cigarette burns, or unusual self-marking may represent unconscious sequelae of SRA beliefs that are behaviorally reenacted.

Other Symptoms

A variety of other unexplained emotional and behavioral disorders that are unresponsive to treatment may be present, including eating, sleep, depressive, and anxiety disorders. Cult-related activities may be presented through the patients' journals or artwork.

Credibility of Patient Accounts

Several factors common to a highly hypnotizable dissociative population contribute to diagnostic complexity.

The credibility of patient accounts may be contaminated by confabulation, malingering, false memory, mass hysteria (Colligan et al. 1982; Markush 1973), the inherent subjectivity of memory, and memory distortions retrieved through hypnosis (American Medical Association 1985; Greaves 1992; Orne 1979; Pettinati 1988;

Young 1992). Accurate recognition and diagnosis also may be confused by iatrogenic influences.

Patients who participate in therapy or recovery groups with other survivors, or who read the burgeoning literature of survivor stories, are susceptible to *source amnesia*. This phenomenon is characterized by a patient's internalizing information about the experience of another person and subsequently forgetting the original source of the information. When the information is recalled, it is perceived by the patient as his or her own experience and is presented as the patient's own reality. Hypnotizable subjects are particularly prone to this form of distortion (Orne 1979; Pettinati 1988).

At present, clinicians lack any measurable or scientific means to distinguish reports that possibly reflect relatively accurate historical accounts from those that have been fantasized, absorbed, confabulated, malingered, suggested, or otherwise created. In the absence of validation from external sources or law enforcement, therapists may need to proceed in a state of ambiguity about historical accuracy while allowing patients to work through the material within their belief systems.

The therapist must remain empathic to the patient's own reality and allow the patient to arrive at his or her own truth. Initial patient accounts often change and reorganize during treatment as dissociated information held in altered states is reintegrated into the patient's overall conscious memory.

In many ways, patients diagnosed as having SRA, when dissociative features predominate, are similar to those who have MPD/DID and related conditions (Braun 1986; Putnam 1989; Ross 1989). Generally, patients are unaware that they have dissociated memories relating to ritual abuse. They may present with any number of symptoms, including depression, anxiety disorders, adjustment disorders, or behavioral problems. They may come into treatment specifically to work through childhood incest. They also may be misdiagnosed as schizophrenic, borderline, bipolar, or delusional.

However, increasing numbers of patients are seeking treatment directly for the emotional sequelae of SRA components of their histories. Until the last few years, patients who knew or suspected SRA tended to be highly secretive about disclosing experiences, even to other survivors. As survivor networks have increased and information has become more available through conferences and lay media, some patients have begun describing their experiences and actively reenacting ritual abuse scenarios during therapy.

For example, a patient diagnosed with SRA presented herself for hospital admission dressed in black, with dyed black hair and black eye shadow. She became histrionic immediately on arriving at the hospital. She identified herself as the high priestess and became verbally and physically assaultive. Several vials of blood were discovered in her luggage. Such histrionic behaviors by cultic alters reflect a change in population profiles. Some patients now demand acceptance of their accounts even before they, themselves, accept them. This demand is in stark contrast to prior experiences when patients were unaware of SRA and denied the reality of images that emerged during treatment.

Treatment Issues

When a patient with a dissociative condition reports SRA, the therapist proceeds with a treatment plan incorporating principles known to be pertinent to abused individuals with posttraumatic stress sequelae and dissociative disorders.

Preparing for Treatment

Before treatment begins, it is essential to assess the patient's external and internal resources. These resources include supportive relationships, a therapist, and access to sufficient financial resources to sustain treatment. It is also important to assess any circumstances in the patient's life (such as a pregnancy, new job, or divorce) that might warrant postponing treatment. Discovery of dissociated material can be intensely disorganizing and volatile.

Patients retrieving dissociated material will experience highly charged states of arousal, flashbacks, panic, and emotional, physical, and physiological reactions similar to those present when the trauma occurred. Therefore, before intensive treatment is begun, patients should be taught as many skills in regulating their emotions as possible. Therapists can teach relaxation, guided imagery, and self-hypnotic techniques. Patients may use exercise programs, music, hobbies, and support groups. Journal writing is an excellent therapeutic adjunct, and the book *Journal to the Self* (Adams 1990a) is recommended as a resource for both patients and therapists. Artwork, movement, and other expressive outlets also can be encouraged. Using a sand tray for expressing inner conflict has been helpful (Sachs 1990). Leisure activities and hobbies can be encouraged to ease excessive states of arousal.

A list of these activities should be prepared in advance, so the patient can refer to it when overwhelmed and when stress threatens clear thinking. Patients often experience stress as an all-or-nothing crisis that is life threatening and endless. They must be concretely taught the difference between small problems and significant crises.

An informed consent should be given regarding the difficulties and potential disorganizing effects of long-term treatment.

Clear therapeutic boundaries and limits must be established at the beginning of treatment. These limits include understanding the therapeutic relationship, the patient's role in treatment, agreements regarding length and frequency of sessions, what constitutes an emergency, under what circumstances the therapist may be paged or telephoned, agreements regarding medication, and other limits the therapist may wish to communicate. Many therapists who are new to the treatment of MPD/DID and the SRA phenomenon establish unrealistically loose boundaries and respond to countertransferential pressures to gratify their patients' demands. Although excessive rigidity is not recommended, excessive gratification often reinforces patients' unrealistic fantasies that other people, the environment, or society will adapt to meet their needs.

Therapeutic interventions such as contracting for safety, closing the system, or developing an inner safe place (Kluft 1982, 1983; Putnam 1989; Young 1992) are resources that should be put in place before efforts toward recall are begun. These structures help build containment and pacing for subsequent stages of treatment.

Because of the pitfalls in memory retrieval and the multiple ways memory can be distorted, confused, absorbed, fabricated, and spread, the patient should be thoroughly informed. A consent form can be provided to educate the patient about problems working with dissociative states and issues pertinent to hypnosis. Even if hypnosis is not formally used, patients are often in and out of trance states, and suggestion may be equally influential with highly hypnotizable subjects. For examples of informed consent, see Appendixes A and B to this chapter.

Early Treatment Issues

Early treatment issues for an SRA patient are similar to those described for an MPD/DID patient (Braun 1986; Putnam 1989; Ross 1989), with the added caution that when SRA is suspected at the onset, the therapist needs to be particularly careful that the patient is not flooded with images of abuse before she or he has been properly prepared (Fine 1991).

Treatment proceeds by identifying the various altered states and dissociative patterns and then developing alliances with the patient in these states. Although these personality states are experienced as concrete and literally real by the patient and are often hidden from her or him through amnesic barriers, they actually reflect defensive dissociative structures evolved from childhood. Many therapists can be led astray by concentrating excessively on these patterns and personalities instead of resolving the information they contain. Generally, it is unwise to attempt to manipulate alter personalities into compliance or to point out the illogic of the system or organization of dissociated internal states and alters. Dissociative states are not developed for reasons of logic but because they are effective in defending against memories of abuse, avoiding hyperarousal, protecting, and surviving an intolerable childhood environment.

The key early issues of treatment are establishing trust and creating an alliance with presenting alters, understanding dissociative functions and defensive patterns, avoiding iatrogenic contamination, and correcting major cognitive distortions.

Establishing trust and creating an alliance with presenting alters. Survivors with SRA beliefs have significant problems developing trusting relationships and will repeatedly test the therapist through acting out, presenting crises, demanding extra time, and bending established limits. It is crucial that the therapist recognize and acknowledge the patient's fears, maintain healthy boundaries and limits, and interpret the acting out as a means to avoid a longed-for connection. Until the alliance is firmly established, the therapist can expect tentative movements toward relating, followed by fearful retreats into behavioral avoidance, acting out, defensive dissociations, projection, or externalizing the problem to others. Hostile or persecutory alters can be understood and accepted as efforts to ensure survival.

Understanding dissociative functions and defensive patterns. SRA patients live in a world of hidden memories and complicated dissociated structures. These structures are usually poorly known to patients and contain dissociated information that in time must be assimilated into their overall awareness. Despite amnesia for their own memories and dissociated states, patients have strong attachment needs that often exceed their capacity to bond in relationships. Automatic dissociative behaviors often can be understood as efforts to avoid a growing external alliance.

The therapist may be subject to a variety of projections or projective identifications. Patients commonly accuse therapists of being untrustworthy, having harmful intent, or otherwise acting like perpetrators. These projections often can be broken up by helping the patient see how the irrational fears reenact a time when as a small child she or he felt betrayed by others.

Reenactments can occur not only externally, with therapists and others in supportive roles, but also internally, within the patient. For example, one woman felt pursued by her parents and had taken precautions to make sure no one in her family knew where she lived. In a dissociated state, she ordered flowers and had them delivered to herself, supposedly from her parents. She was in a state of panic until she was able to recognize the internal reenactment.

Avoiding iatrogenic contamination. The therapist must be constantly alert to the problem of iatrogenically introduced material because dissociative patients are prone to suspend critical judgment and accept suggestion as truth, both in and out of hypnotic trance.

Correcting major cognitive distortions. When traumatic experiences are dissociated, the cognitive forms present at the time of trauma are dissociated in the same distorted form. This dissociation leads to a wide variety of cognitive distortions, including all-or-none thinking, egocentricity, assuming blame or fault, errant cause-and-effect assessment, and over- or undergeneralization of stimuli (Fine 1988, 1991). For example, a patient blamed herself for times when the therapist was unavoidably detained or canceled an appointment due to illness.

A much healthier synthesis of the trauma and its meaning becomes possible when cognitive distortions are recognized with the patient and corrected. Patients may need concrete education in these areas, including the notion that crises are not always emergencies and do have endpoints.

Intermediate Issues in Treatment

During the lengthy and often difficult intermediate phase, dissociative defenses dissolve, and most of the work toward resolving trauma is accomplished. There is continued work on the relationship with the therapist and others in the real world, approaching and working through traumatic memories, shifting away from automatic dissociation, organizing the traumatic material, further correcting cognitive distortion, and moving toward integration as alter personalities yield their information. Abreaction is frequently encountered as material is reactivated and vividly reexperienced. A variety of ancillary therapeutic techniques are helpful here, as are the previously learned containment skills.

Expressive arts therapies. Expressive arts therapies such as art, dance and movement, and journal therapy are useful treatment adjuncts. Art therapy allows expressive drawing, painting, sculpture, or collage to reveal visual content of memories, some of which may not yet have been verbalized. Through art therapy, the patient can bypass prohibitions against telling. Art is also useful in recognizing emerging themes and providing creative release.

Dance and movement therapy can show a great deal about tension states and chronic patterns of holding physical energy. It allows the patient to recognize body image problems and physical inhibitions and provides physical release.

Journaling, also known as journal therapy (Adams 1990a, 1990b, 1991), can help patients retrieve dissociated material, develop coconsciousness, dialogue among parts of the system (pattern or organization of internal states), and contain painful memories. The written record of the healing process can be reviewed at key stages of therapy and can serve both as a testament to the progress being made and as a bridge into new learned behaviors (Adams 1990b).

Recreational therapy encourages the patient to investigate new leisure and socialization skills and helps the patient overcome blocks to appropriate pleasure.

Self-hypnosis. Self-hypnotic techniques allow the patient to self-regulate and manage overstimulation through imagery and relaxation.

Finger signals. Ideomotor (finger) signaling in a light trance state is a helpful technique to access altered states and quickly gather information that is not yet in conscious awareness. The therapist can teach the patient how to answer yes/no questions using simple finger signals such as moving the index finger for "yes," moving the thumb for "no," rolling the hand outward for "I don't know," and raising a palm up for "stop." The hands are kept in the lap. This ideomotor signaling technique is useful for assessing safety, negotiating contracts, and asking for information from internal alter personalities. It is also a useful device for communicating with acting-out or destructive altered states while keeping them inside.

The caution required in working with hypnosis and memory cannot be overemphasized. Skillful use of hypnosis can be an enormous treatment adjunct, but the risks of error and iatrogenic suggestion are omnipresent. It is recommended that therapists who work with SRA patients take formal hypnosis training with reputable teachers (Fraser 1991; Hammond 1992).

Later Issues in Treatment

Issues specific to SRA present predictable obstacles to treatment and arise most prominently in middle and late phases of therapy.

Yielding forbidden information is accompanied by the emergence of a variety of alters related to the SRA experience, the most difficult of which are satanic or cultic alters emerging to punish the patient for breaking the code of secrecy. As cultic alters and their associated traumas surface, the whole system or organization of internal states can be seen to modify, pull together, and move toward fusion.

Often, much therapeutic attention is directed to programs, triggers, cues, and a variety of deceptive practices that were reportedly used by cult members (for further discussion, see pp. 80–83). These techniques were allegedly used to gain control of the patient's thinking as a child. As dissociative barriers break down, adult perspectives begin to develop and deceptions begin to be recognized.

When dangerous alters or frightening memories surface, helping personalities can be engaged to maintain safety between sessions. For example, when working with a particularly painful or disorganizing memory, the therapist may ask for a part of the system of dissociated internal states to act as an organizer of the information or as a protector to prevent escalation or loss of control. It is important to pace the treatment to incorporate periods of rest and consolidation.

Treating Satanic Alters

Alter personality states can be likened to information storage banks that contain unassimilated traumatic information. Data are stored in their raw form, with their heightened affect and kinesthetic qualities intact and their contents highly disorganized. As information is retrieved and integrated into the patient's overall knowledge base, personalities begin integrating, and sources of reenactment behaviors become available for change.

The key for therapists is to focus on organizing or reorganizing the past and its archaic meaning rather than focusing on manipulating the personalities. Although it is to be expected that the patient will experience herself or himself as many discrete parts, it is imperative that the therapist constantly be aware that the patient is a single traumatized adult. This is especially true when working with hostile or satanic alters.

As patients begin to talk about SRA in therapy, self-abusive, acting-out personality states usually appear to protest or stop the disclosures. These alters often function as, or are identified with, satanic or cultic beliefs. It is our experience that satanic or cultic alters do not reflect literal evil entities; rather, these alters represent dissociated personality states with the same defensive functions as any other altered state.

Such dissociated states are experienced as behaviors learned after prolonged conditioning. Forming satanic alters may also reflect the patient's identification with the aggressor. The patient may have attempted mastery by creating internal entities as strong and powerful as her or his perpetrators. In some cases, so-called cultic alters are reported to be fostered deliberately by perpetrators who indoctrinate through force or torture. This development of satanic or cultic alters can be better understood as the patient's yielding to, complying with, and identifying with the perpetrator in an effort to stop the abuse.

Regardless of the etiology, the evolution and maintenance of satanic alters supposedly reflect coerced or spontaneous identifications with those in power and are an aspect of the patient's vulnerability.

Hostile or oppositional alters seem to be part of the total memory package, and their appearance can be regarded as an expected developmental stage in treatment. When these oppositional personality states present as satanic or cultic alters, they will appear to uphold and comply with the prevailing culture of the cult's secrecy, power, and group beliefs. These alters perceive themselves to be at risk by outside or inside cult figures if they fail to enforce secrecy.

Although the therapeutic alliance is more difficult when altered states present as hostile, vitriolic, or oppositional, the alliance nonetheless remains the first task in dealing with satanic alters. Once the alliance is established, the therapist can explore the dissociative barriers to the trauma that are reported to have formed the satanic states.

In most instances, satanic alters indicate a singularly linear and concrete line of thinking and have little capacity to reflect on the possibility that they have choices or that they may be amnesic for their own abuse. They understand power in hierarchical terms only and do not recognize that self-empowerment reflects the capacity to make healthy choices. Satanic alters cannot grasp that adhering to what a cult taught them to believe is not an issue of power but one of servitude and compliance.

Gradually recognizing their own traumatic origin frees satanic alters to recognize how few choices they had in their own beliefs and behaviors. Recollecting their own trauma and restoring their freedom of choice are powerful tools that reduce the antagonism of these satanic alters and allow them to change their identification as satanic alters. This change also reflects the increased awareness of sequestered information about their own intimidation, decreasing the need for dissociative defenses and allowing freedom for self-discovery and movement toward cohesive functioning.

It is often necessary to educate satanic alters that choice is a form of personal power. Satanic alters need reassurance that life is not a struggle for power through aggression. They need to learn that as they make their own choices instead of adhering to their past patterns of obedience, life becomes fuller, freer, and more powerful. The therapist can interpret to the patient that, despite the possibility that the alters might have enjoyed destructive activities, the satanic states have served a helping function by preserving the patient's silence at a time when silence was equated with survival. This notion of satanic alters as helpers is usually unrecognized by the patient and can be leverage to stop fighting their emergence and start learning about them with more acceptance.

Satanic alters often experience themselves as emotionless, unfeeling, or robotic. It is helpful to point out that hostility and anger are emotions and that they may barricade any broader range of feelings present beneath the dissociation. Awareness of a broader range of feelings often helps satanic alters understand their limited functioning.

All dissociative states are part of a single person with one experiential world shared by all. As memories, feelings, and somatic responses push through, satanic alters begin to integrate into that experiential world.

Programs, Triggers, and Cues

SRA patients report phenomena couched in cultlike descriptions of programs, triggers, and cues. These phenomena are believed in by patients and described concretely. The reports may become increasingly bizarre and complex during treatment, suggesting the possibility of confabulated elaboration. A *program*, for example, could be defined as a behavior taught through intimidation and torture to be enacted at a future date or in response to a signal or cue. Patients might report that they were programmed for self-mutilation, suicide, or return to cult life on a birthday, or some other particular behavior, in response to some signal, such as having told secrets in therapy. Because programs are dissociated, patients' experiences are frequently felt as domination by external, rather than internal, forces that cannot be resisted. Patients believe that they are controlled, pursued, or stalked by cult members or supernatural forces.

In most instances, patients are responding to inner states that are confused as external realities. They are simply not aware that the pressure is an internal reenactment that could be resisted. This confusion can lead to terror and a sense of extreme urgency, which unfortunately can affect the therapist's judgment as well. Therapists may feel compelled to intervene with concrete countertransference responses such as prolonged sessions, direct nurturance, providing shelter, or helping the patient relocate to another city or state. As treatment progresses, differences between reenactment and external reality become clarified, and patients begin to modify their behaviors.

A *cue* is a verbal, visual, or auditory signal that initiates a programmed behavior. It is a specific stimulus that provokes a specified response. A *trigger*, on the other hand, reflects a generalized stimulus that inadvertently acts like a cue. A trigger also can be anything that stimulates a frightening image, memory, or emotional response.

This language, used by patients and therapists, casts a sociopolitical shadow on treatment that departs from psychological frames of reference. The language tends to distract both therapists and patients into thinking that they may be dealing with immovable, fixed programs or patterns that have been instilled in some immutable way. This way of thinking leads to a mistaken assumption that the patient may be hardwired to respond in some predetermined way when in fact cognitive states of programs are broken all the time as patients come into treatment, make behavioral changes, make dissociative shifts, and start healing.

For example, patients may describe the pairing of torture or punishment with instructions to suicide if certain secrets were told. Later, if patients tell of abuse, they feel a pressure to hurt themselves. Patients may define this as programming when in fact it can be seen psychologically as conditioning with negative reinforcement.

Substituting language, such as "What did you learn from that?" returns therapy to a psychological frame of reference. The languages of behavior modification, learning theory, and psychodynamics reduce the sense that the patient is a robot and change is impossible. Although it is a gradual process, awareness of cognitive conditioning helps patients recognize the source of the impulse and that it is within their ability to respond differently. As patients respond differently to stimuli, behavioral extinction can occur that may even generalize to other behaviors.

Although patients may continue to use this language, therapists should remain aware of the risk of becoming caught up in their patients' way of thinking, which often includes impossibility, hopelessness, and chaos. Reframing patients' concepts goes a long way toward reducing the excessive mystique of mind control.

Deceptive Practices

Deceptive practices by adults or cult members may be key contributors to memory distortion and are increasingly reported by patients as dissociative barriers are permeated and integration proceeds. It is easy to deceive children when they are in chronic states of fatigue, terror, pain, and confusion. Deceptions commonly reported by SRA survivors produce magical illusions that leave children with lasting impressions that they are dealing with powerful supernatural forces purporting to arise from satanic power and are thus impossible to escape. Patients then become increasingly certain that powers beyond their control can watch them, monitor their thoughts, and track them down should they deviate from cult expectations.

For example, a patient reported being raped by Satan. She knew it was Satan because of his bright red face, long fingernails, horns, and cape. She was asked if anyone inside could provide additional details or saw the event differently. Another personality then announced that the fingernails and horns were fake, the face was merely painted red, and the cape was wrinkled. This puzzled her, as she knew a real Satan wouldn't have a wrinkled cape. She was then able to recognize the voice as one of her father's friends. Subsequently, the patient could see other deceptive episodes.

Another woman recalled being so tightly encircled by robed adults that other children could not witness actual events. A knife was raised and appeared to stab her while red liquid was thrown over her. She was given a sedative by injection. When she awoke, she found herself in the woods with one of the robed men. He sat under a tree smoking a cigarette until he saw her wake up. The man then returned her to the group, where the adults feigned astonishment and praised the power of Satan that he had restored her life.

A non-MPD/DID patient with reasonably good access to organized recall reported that as a teenager she accompanied her father, an engineer and former theater technician, as he staged illusions at satanic meeting sites where the father was allegedly a cult member and the patient a victim of SRA.

These subjective reports are increasingly common. Discovering deceptions has a profound clinical implication. Once patients see they might have been deceived in one way, all personalities are more open to new interpretations of their experiences. They are more willing and able to see that their memories are suggesting they were abused by sadistic people, not powerful deities that cannot be challenged. They can look for other ways they were deceived, including cult teachings.

Pharmacological Approaches

There is no specific medication for SRA or MPD/DID, and no systematic studies have been reported. Therefore, pharmacological treatment should be guided by common sense and directed toward specific symptoms. Loewenstein (1991) and Braun (1990; see also Chapter 8, in this volume) provide good discussions of pharmacological interventions.

Medication regimens should be as simple as possible and discontinued if key symptoms do not improve. It is important to assess whether the symptom appears to pervade most of the dissociative system or whether it is specific to certain dissociative states. As a general guideline, a symptom complex should not be medicated unless it is widespread throughout the system.

The pharmacological approach remains empirical. Because the therapist is essentially dealing with PTSD, the literature on psychopharmacology in PTSD remains the best guide. The traditional medications used for these conditions consist of tricyclic antidepressants; selective serotonin reuptake inhibitors (SSRIs); anxiolytics such as diazepam, lorazepam, chlordiazepoxide, or alprazolam; monoamine oxidase inhibitors (MAOIs); and trials of carbamazepine or valproic acid as mood stabilizers when other regimens do not provide results. With occasional exceptions, antipsychotics are not helpful and may produce further symptoms of dissociation and disconnection. Clonazepam has shown some promise (Loewenstein 1988).

For overwhelming anxiety and flashbacks, anxiolytics are appropriate. Increased dosages may be necessary so that the patient can function well enough to proceed in therapy. Longer-acting agents provide more stable levels and are thus preferable. Loewenstein (1991) reports that clonazepam has been helpful with PTSD symptoms. Many patients in our caseload also have responded well to this regimen.

Depression is such a common symptom that when it is pervasive throughout the dissociated states, antidepressant regimens are indicated to free the patient's constricted affect and allow work to progress. SSRIs, tricyclics, and MAOIs have all been used effectively (Braun, Chapter 8, in this volume; Loewenstein 1991; van der Kolk 1987).

Any drug for which there exists the possibility of psychological or physiological dependence must be monitored closely and discontinued if symptoms are not significantly improved. Patients should be encouraged to develop tolerance for a certain level of anxiety. Avoid narcotic medications whenever possible in the treatment of memory-related or somatic pain.

However, caution is necessary in order not to overlook bona fide illnesses that may appear psychosomatic. For patients who have long periods of hyperarousal, antianxiety agents should be administered in a dosage that is calming but not overly sedating. The ideal dosage allows processing of material without so much sedation that the material is suppressed or cannot be assimilated.

Recent Trends in Treatment

In recent years, new reports and beliefs about memories and mind control, as well as new therapeutic approaches, have introduced additional treatment considerations.

False Memory Syndrome

Overreliance on the accuracy of dissociated memory has become the subject of much debate. Information retrieved from a given dissociated state is only part of a whole story, and early accounts reported by patients are almost always changed or clarified as dissociative barriers are permeated and additional information is brought into awareness. Prematurely validating information produced by patients in dissociated states has led to a new social backlash accusing therapists of creating false ideas by validating unsupported information.

In March 1992, the False Memory Syndrome Foundation was organized in Pennsylvania, primarily by families accused of incest and abuse by their adult children (Orange 1993). This group alleges that some therapists comply with or validate confabulated memories or even suggest memories to patients, leading to premature acceptance of this information as true by both patients and therapists. Litigations against therapists by family members alleging a false memory syndrome should be a reminder that in any patient's treatment, therapists must remain therapists and not interpreters of truth, which comes only with independent documentation.

In any therapy, much of what the therapist hears is a mixture of truth, distortion, and fantasy (Orne 1979; Pettinati 1988; Young 1988, 1992). Obligations of the therapist are not the same as the obligations of social services or law enforcement agencies. It is not always possible for the therapist to assume the role of investigator or protector. The therapist's obligations include understanding the meaning of patients' beliefs, interpreting for patients how these beliefs impact their lives, and resolving the residuals of trauma in the present. Both patients and therapists must tolerate ambiguity. Additionally, therapists must balance uncertain historical under- standing with treatment aimed at empowerment, relatedness, and correction of developmental deficits, and patients must examine the meaning of their own experiences. In their treatment, patients should be encouraged to validate bizarre memories if they can and should have an understanding of the pitfalls of memory.

Eye Movement Desensitization Reprocessing

Eye movement desensitization reprocessing (EMDR), a new meth- od for working with trauma patients, was developed by Shapiro (1989a, 1989b, 1995). Among incest patients and veterans with PTSD, she found that incorporating saccadic eye movements simi- lar to those seen in rapid eye movement sleep produced dramatic lasting results in one or two sessions. The application of EMDR has spread in treating a variety of symptom complexes, including trauma associated with MPD/DID and patients reporting SRA (Fenstermaker 1993; Young 1994). A number of patients in our caseload were treated with EMDR, with favorable results in some cases and resistance to the treatment in others.

One patient had sensed herself for some time to be on the verge of integrating her dissociated states. Following EMDR, a massive dissolution of amnesia occurred with release of memories. She was confused and disoriented for several days. However, when she re- covered, the patient reported markedly enhanced awareness and a feeling of rapid resolution of her traumatic memory. The patient stated that overall she felt the procedure helped her.

Patients who respond positively to EMDR state that they feel the work progresses faster and is processed differently than tradi- tional treatment approaches. Those who resist the procedure gen- erally fear uncovering too much material at once. One patient consulting the authors stated that EMDR was helpful but her thera- pist had not allowed sufficient processing time before moving on. This patient stopped formal EMDR but continued work with eye movement at her own pace at home.

EMDR may find a place in the treatment of those with memories of SRA. Appropriate target symptoms and approaches should be assessed. Because the theoretical underpinnings of EMDR are still speculative, controlled trials with techniques such as fractionated hypnotic abreactions should be examined. Using EMDR to treat the SRA population should be limited to therapists experienced and trained to work with both EMDR and SRA, and a cautious approach with a fully informed consent should be instituted until further study illuminates the role EMDR has in resolving ritual trauma. Potential problems likely to affect how EMDR is ultimately used in treating SRA include the massive amount of material released and lack of organization or integration of the material. EMDR is no substitute for good clinical judgment.

Conclusion

SRA perpetrated by satanic cults is increasingly reported among patient populations who display complex dissociative and other posttraumatic features of severe abuse syndromes. Alternative explanations offered by the professional community treating such patients include psychogenic hysteria, suggestibility, confabulation, and absorption.

The case for SRA is hampered by a lack of confirming evidence from social services or law enforcement agencies, as well as by increasingly bizarre reports from patients. Therapists sometimes confuse high levels of emotional intensity with historical accuracy and must learn how to accept information at face value without overinvesting in its literal truth.

Intense abreactive experiences by highly hypnotizable subjects can lead them to believe with absolute certainty in events that never transpired (Pettinati 1988). Memory is at best an imperfect function, and we have no instruments to differentiate accurate recall from distortion (American Medical Association 1985; Orne 1979; Pettinati 1988; Young 1992). Any memory is a mixture of truth, distortion, and confabulation. Despite this fact, even suggestible people can portray historical events accurately, and the wise therapist will judge nothing prematurely while tolerating the ambiguity inherent in SRA.

The most effective therapists develop treatment strategies to work within the context of their patients' realities. These therapists meet patients at their present levels of understanding and gradually help them explore how dissociated trauma has impacted their behaviors, reality testing, choice making, and capacities for intimacy and self-esteem. Treatment can free up the massive amounts of emotional energy consumed by maintaining dissociative states and other defensive structures. This emotional energy can be redirected into learning how to share intimate relationships instead of remaining connected to alters and their memories of the past.

As treatment progresses, internalized prohibitions against disclosure often result in behavioral escalation and full-blown posttraumatic stress syndromes, including self-abusive behaviors, abreactions, and chronic traumatic states. Treatment thus begins with ego-strengthening and self-management skills.

The gradual lifting of dissociative barriers allows access to sequestered information that, once in conscious awareness, can be assimilated, worked through, and integrated.

It is imperative that therapists not be pulled from a therapeutic stance by entering into patients' pathological experiences. Endless abreactive sessions do not lead to change; they only reenact trauma and perpetuate patients' victimization. Patients are often so compelling in the intensity and urgency of their reports that therapists are drawn into ongoing crisis management, and no time is left for interpreting the experience in the present. Losing therapeutic perspective and leverage often leads a therapist into overinvolvement, burnout, secondary PTSD symptoms, and other countertransference responses. When therapy is realigned and boundaries are reinstated, the patient can begin to assume responsibility in treatment and work toward individual empowerment, even without absolute knowledge of the past.

Postdiscovery and postintegration phases are characterized by identity and existential crises in which patients question why they survived, what the future holds, who they are as single personalities, and what meaning their lives intrinsically offer. They must learn to live, grieve, trust, risk, err, connect, and relate without dissociation. Issues of deeper meaning and purpose are explored. It is often a time of spiritual crisis and emergence. Although these existential dilemmas and crises echo throughout treatment, they reverberate at the postintegration phase. A new cycle of therapy begins, and the significance, meaning, and validity of the experience can often be addressed.

Patients revealing memories of ritual abuse can be successfully treated, although emotional scars will remain. Many factors contribute to a good prognosis. For the patient, they include motivation, basic ego strength, reasonably good impulse control, capacity for hope, and future orientation. For the therapist, they include a humane willingness to join empathically in the patient's experience without aligning with the pathology.

References

Adams K: Journal to the Self: 22 Paths to Personal Growth. New York, Warner Books, 1990a

Adams K: The 79¢ Therapist: The Journal as Psychological Toolbox (Audiotape No JO–1). Boulder, CO, Sounds True, 1990b

Adams K (ed): Journals Quick and Easy. Arvada, CO, The Center for Journal Therapy, 1991

American Medical Association Council on Scientific Affairs: Council report: scientific status of refreshing recollection by the use of hypnosis. JAMA 253:1918–1923, 1985

American Psychiatric Association: Diagnostic and Statistical Manual of Mental Disorders, 3rd Edition, Revised. Washington, DC, American Psychiatric Association, 1987

American Psychiatric Association: Diagnostic and Statistical Manual of Mental Disorders, 4th Edition. Washington, DC, American Psychiatric Association, 1994

Braun BG (ed): Treatment of Multiple Personality Disorder. Washington, DC, American Psychiatric Press, 1986

Braun BG: Unusual medication regimens in the treatment of dissociative disorder patients, I: noradrenergic agents. Dissociation 3:144–150, 1990

Colligan MJ, Pennebaker JW, Murphey LR (eds): Mass Psychogenic Amnesia: A Social Psychological Analysis. Hillsdale, NJ, Lawrence Erlbaum, 1982

Fenstermaker D: Multiple personality disorder. Paper presented at the Second Annual Eye Movement Desensitization Reprocessing Conference on Research and Clinical Applications, Sunnyvale, CA, March 1993

Fine CG: Thoughts on the cognitive perceptual substrates of multiple per-
    sonality disorders. Dissociation 1:5–10, 1988
Fine CG: Treatment stabilization and crisis intervention: pacing the ther-
    apy of the multiple personality patient. Psychiatr Clin North Am
    14:661–675, 1991
Fraser GA: Satanic ritual abuse: a cause of multiple personality disorder.
    Journal of Child and Youth Care (special issue):55–66, 1990
Fraser GA: The dissociative table technique: a strategy for working with
    ego states in dissociative disorders and ego-state therapy. Dissociation
    4:205–213, 1991
Ganaway GK: Historical truth versus narrative truth: clarifying the role
    of exogenous trauma in the etiology of multiple personality disorder
    and its variance. Dissociation 2:205–220, 1989
Ganaway GK: Satanic ritual abuse: critical issues and alternative hy-
    potheses. Panel presentation at the Seventh International Confer-
    ence on Multiple Personality/Dissociative States, Chicago, IL,
    November 1990
Gardner RA: True and False Accusations of Child Sex Abuse. Longwood,
    NJ, Creative Therapeutics, 1992
Gould C: Satanic ritual abuse: child victims, adult survivors, system re-
    sponse. California Psychologist 3:76–92, 1987
Gould C: Diagnosis and treatment of ritually abused children, in Out of
    Darkness: Exploring Satanism and Ritual Abuse. Edited by Sakheim
    DK, Devine SE. New York, Lexington Books, 1992, pp 247–248
Greaves GB: Alternative hypotheses regarding claims of satanic cult ac-
    tivity: a critical analysis, in Out of Darkness: Exploring Satanism and
    Ritual Abuse. Edited by Sakheim DK, Devine SE. New York, Lexington
    Books, 1992, pp 45–72
Hammond C: Training and treatment. Paper presented at the Fourth An-
    nual Eastern Regional Conference on Abuse and Multiple Personality
    Disorder, Alexandria, VA, June 1992
Hill S, Goodwin J: Satanism: similarities between patient accounts and
    pre-Inquisition historical sources. Dissociation 2:39–44, 1989
Jones DPH: Ritualism and child sexual abuse. Child Abuse Negl 15:163–
    170, 1991
Jonker F, Jonker-Bakker P: Commentary: experiences with ritualistic child
    sexual abuse: a case study from the Netherlands. Child Abuse Negl
    15:191–196, 1991
Kelly SJ: Ritualistic abuse of children: dynamics and impact. Cultic Studies
    Journal 2:228–236, 1988

Kelly SJ: Stress responses of children to sexual abuse and ritualistic abuse in day care centers. Journal of Interpersonal Violence 4:501–513, 1989

Kinscherff R, Barnum R: Child forensic evaluation and claims of ritual abuse or satanic activity: a critical analysis, in Out of Darkness: Exploring Satanism and Ritual Abuse. Edited by Sakheim DK, Devine SE. New York, Lexington Books, 1992, pp 73–108

Kluft RP: Hypnotherapeutic crisis intervention in multiple personality. Am J Clin Hypn 24:73–83, 1982

Kluft RP: Varieties of hypnotic interventions in the treatment of multiple personality. Am J Clin Hypn 26:230–240, 1983

Kluft RP: Editorial: reflections on allegations of ritual abuse. Dissociation 2:191–193, 1989

Lanning KV: Commentary: ritual abuse: a law enforcement view or perspective. Child Abuse Negl 15:171–174, 1991

Lanning KV: A law enforcement perspective on allegations of ritual abuse, in Out of Darkness: Exploring Satanism and Ritual Abuse. Edited by Sakheim DK, Devine SE. New York, Lexington Books, 1992, pp 109–146

Loewenstein RJ: Open trial of clonazepam in the treatment of posttraumatic stress symptoms in multiple personality disorder. Dissociation 1:3–12, 1988

Loewenstein RJ: Rational psychopharmacology in the treatment of multiple personality disorder. Psychiatr Clin North Am 14:721–740, 1991

Loftus E, Ketcham K: The Myth of Repressed Memory. New York, St. Martin's Press, 1994

Markush RE: Mental epidemics. Public Health Review 2:353–442, 1973

Mulhern S: Satanic ritual abuse: critical issues and alternative hypotheses. Panel presentation at the Seventh International Conference on Multiple Personality/Dissociative States, Chicago, IL, November 1990

Mulhern S: Embodied alternative identities: bearing witness to a world that might have been. Psychiatr Clin North Am 14:769–786, 1991

Noll R: Satanism, UFO abductions, historians and clinicians: those who do not remember the past. Dissociation 2:251–253, 1989

Noll R: Satanic ritual abuse: critical issues and alternative hypotheses. Panel presentation at the Seventh International Conference on Multiple Personality/Dissociative States, Chicago, IL, November 1990

Ofshe R, Watters E: Making Monsters. New York, Scribners, 1994

Orange LM: Long-Delayed Memories of Abuse: True Recall or Artifact of Therapy. Rockville, MD, International Medical News Group, 1993

Orne MT: The use and misuse of hypnosis in court. Int J Clin Exp Hypn 27:311–341, 1979

Pettinati HM (ed): Hypnosis and Memory. New York, Guilford, 1988

Putnam FW: Dissociation as a response to extreme trauma, in Childhood Antecedents of Multiple Personality. Edited by Kluft RP. Washington, DC, American Psychiatric Press, 1985, pp 65–97

Putnam FW: Diagnosis and Treatment of Multiple Personality Disorder. New York, Guilford, 1989

Putnam FW: Satanic ritual abuse: critical issues and alternative hypotheses. Panel presentation at the Seventh International Conference on Multiple Personality/Dissociative States. Chicago, IL, November 1990

Putnam FW: Commentary: the satanic ritual abuse controversy. Child Abuse Negl 15:175–180, 1991

Richardson JT, Best J, Bromley DG: The Satanism Scare. New York, Aldine de Gruyter, 1991

Ross CA: Multiple Personality Disorder Diagnosis, Clinical Features, and Treatment. New York, Wiley, 1989

Sachs RG: Sandtray technique in the treatment of dissociative disorders: recommendations for occupational therapists. Am J Occup Ther 44:1045–1047, 1990

Sakheim DK, Devine SE: Out of Darkness: Exploring Satanism and Ritual Abuse. New York, Lexington Books, 1992

Shapiro F: Efficacy of eye movement desensitization procedure in the treatment of traumatic memories. J Trauma Stress 2:199–223, 1989a

Shapiro F: Eye movement desensitization: a new treatment for posttraumatic stress disorder. J Behav Ther Exp Psychiatry 20:211–217, 1989b

Shapiro F: Eye Movement Desensitization and Reprocessing: Basic Principles, Protocols and Procedures. New York, Guilford, 1995

Snow B: Ritualistic child abuse in a neighbourhood setting. Journal of Interpersonal Violence 5:474–487, 1990

Spiegel D: Multiple personality as a posttraumatic stress disorder. Psychiatr Clin North Am 7:101–110, 1984

Spiegel D: Dissociation and hypnosis in posttraumatic stress disorders. J Trauma Stress 1:17–33, 1988

Tennant-Clark CM, Fritz J, Beauvai F: Occult participation: its impact on adolescent development. Adolescence 24:757–772, 1989

Van Benschoten SC: Multiple personality disorder and satanic ritual abuse: the issue of credibility. Dissociation 3:22–30, 1990

van der Kolk BA: Psychological Trauma. Washington, DC, American Psychiatric Press, 1987

Victor J: Satanic Panic: The Creation of a Contemporary Legend. Chicago, IL, Open Court, 1993

Young WC: Observations on fantasy in the formation of multiple personality disorder. Dissociation 1:13–19, 1988

Young WC: Recognition and treatment of survivors reporting ritual abuse, in Out of Darkness: Exploring Satanism and Ritual Abuse. Edited by Sakheim DK, Devine SE. New York, Lexington Books, 1992

Young WC: EMDR treatment of phobia symptoms in multiple personality disorder. Dissociation 7:129–133, 1994

Young WC, Sachs RG, Braun BG, et al: Patients reporting ritual abuse in childhood: a clinical syndrome: report of 37 cases. Child Abuse Negl 15:181–189, 1991

Informed Consent Regarding the Treatment of Traumatic and Dissociative Disorders

This important information about your treatment is provided to help you understand the benefits and potential pitfalls in treating traumatic and dissociative disorders. It is not meant to undermine your personal experience or make light of any work you have done. Rather, it is felt that an informed person will be able to weigh the risks and benefits of treatment and to be aware of problem areas that may have a bearing on your recovery. This information can help you to make the most responsible decisions about your own treatment and to interpret traumatic material that may emerge as you progress.

There are many issues that you need to know about your treatment. Many patients experience a variety of problems in the course of their treatment, including flashbacks, flooding of emotions, overstimulation, nightmares, anxiety and panic attacks, suicidality, self-destructive or angry impulses, depression, increased dissociative behavior, and feelings of disorganization. There may be a need for hospital care at times. Some people may have trouble maintaining employment or have problems with their social and family relationships. It is possible to feel worse before one feels better, and some people may not feel they get better but just feel worse. Others may find they regularly feel better. Your therapy can feel demanding, and it is important that you develop friends, helpful support, activities, and other personal resources to turn to if you are in a crisis and your therapist is not available. These problems can be anticipated and discussed with your therapist.

On the other hand, most people coming into treatment are already having severe symptoms and feel they need to enter treatment because of the problems that they are already facing. In most cases, therapy may be the only way to regain a sense of balance and health. You must decide whether the risks of treatment, even if it turns out not to be helpful, are acceptable if it offers a hope for a happier and more integrated life.

The treatment of traumatic and dissociative disorders is still evolving, and it is not possible to predict what your treatment experience will be. This will also depend upon factors in you and your fit with your therapist.

Ordinarily, your treatment will include a variety of components to help you gain self-control and improve your personal relationships and your functioning in the present. It will address erroneous patterns of thinking, as well as reenactment of old conflicts through your behavior, and will help to resolve the residuals of trauma and abuse. Treatment can take months or years for some and be much briefer for others. There is no way to predict a length of therapy. Hospitalization should be as brief as possible to prevent an interruption of your life.

There are other approaches that are available to you or that can be used simultaneously. These include a variety of traditional psychotherapies, group therapies, cognitive therapy, behavior modification techniques, hypnosis, eye movement desensitization reprocessing (EMDR) or accelerated information processing (AIP), and a variety of medications. Some people feel that treatment makes them feel worse and prefer to stop. You need to discuss your plan with your therapist. Consultations or a second opinion can always be requested if you feel stuck.

The mental health field is presently divided in its beliefs about and understanding of dissociation and the validity of repressed memories retrieved in adulthood or during treatment. On one end of the spectrum are therapists who accept all material as accurate with no independent corroboration, and they may suggest the presence of abuse memories based on symptoms even when memories are absent. On the other end of the spectrum are those who believe that abuse memories are not repressed, that amnesia for severe abuse does not occur, and that abuse memories are implanted by poorly informed therapists in unwitting, naive, or suggestible patients. Given this division, even among many credible professionals, it is exceedingly important to be aware of what we believe so that your treatment leads you to your own conclusions and you are aware of alternative approaches from which to choose. It is hoped that informed decisions and an open mind will give you the best chance to heal.

Studies to date have clearly established the presence of child sexual, physical, and emotional abuse. They have also shown that a variety of adult behaviors and symptoms are correlated with a history of abuse. There are, however, instances where abuse may not always lead to significant disturbance; simultaneously, many symptomatic individuals may not have a history of severe abuse. Reports of memories for abuse do not guarantee its authenticity, nor, on the other hand, does a failure to recall abuse mean that none was present.

Our best understanding at present is that memories of abuse may be accurate, distorted, confabulated, dissociated, repressed from conscious recall, or contaminated by a variety of other factors.

Further, memories of traumatic events may change over time as new information that is repressed or discovered becomes available. For this reason, it is wise to suspend judgment on memories until sufficient time has elapsed to allow the dissociated information to emerge and cognitive distortions to be corrected, so a fuller and more accurate assimilation of retrieved material can be completed and a clearer perspective and meaning of these events can be integrated.

You should know that amnesia for traumatic events and child abuse is a regularly documented finding. What is less well known, and often objected to on the basis of its appearing to reinjure abuse survivors, is the recognition that people can, under a variety of circumstances, appear to remember events that in fact never happened. In other instances, events may have happened quite differently than they are remembered. Even inaccurate recall, however, does not mean that some kind of abuse did not occur.

Inaccurate recollections can, in some instances, be experienced as so real and vivid and can be accompanied by such significant physical sensations or body pain that they are accepted as real memories with absolute conviction.

This is not meant to discount what you know but to permit you the widest possible latitude in reconstructing your life. Memory is a complicated business. Real memory also can be recalled with intensity, vividness, and physical sensations that reflect a representation of the original trauma. This is especially true with repressed memory and particularly in dissociative conditions. In dissociative conditions, the manner in which traumatic material is stored makes this problem especially difficult because accurate, distorted, and inaccurate information can be experienced similarly and believed with the same conviction.

There is no way that professionals can tell with certainty the historical accuracy of any account, and therefore it is important to know that professionals cannot validate the historical truth of any memory. The concern about being unable to validate individuals' accounts of their personal history is presented to help you know the limitations of therapy. Validation is something that must be established with independent corroboration; for instance, you might allow your therapist, if it is appropriate, to contact people in your life directly to attempt to clarify what is true, despite knowing from the literature that there is a pattern of denial in families where abuse has occurred. This contact would be recommended only if it were therapeutically indicated and then only with your written consent.

This information is not meant to discount the impact of your suffering or to suggest that you not discuss the material that emerges in your treatment. Recollections, even in people who inadvertently may have accepted inaccurate information as memories, will continue to have a significant impact on how people organize and think about their lives. These recollections, despite the issue of accuracy, are still what shapes self-esteem, influences behavior, and provides meaning and perspective for people's lives. It is important, however, that you know that severe child abuse is a known fact and that severe trauma can be forgotten and dissociated by many people and in a variety of situations.

There are times when people recall memories of things that have not occurred to them, and more problematic still are those who purposefully will present false memory for their own reasons. A professional therapist has no way of knowing the difference. Therefore, the therapist must help some people who unknowingly report erroneous memory by periodically challenging or trying to understand material in new ways, allowing those people to arrive at different or more accurate formulations about their recollections and the impact these recollections have had.

Professionals have encountered memories they have not believed that subsequently turned out to be true, and similarly they have encountered memories they believed to be true that have turned out not to be. As a result, therapists and patients have had to work together, understanding and tolerating the difficulties in knowing the accuracy or inaccuracy of what emerges in therapy. Your therapist may write or use terms such as *recall, memory, repressed memory, a history of,* and similar terms. In the absence of external corroboration, you, your treatment team, and your therapist are aware that these terms are used for convenience in communicating and not as a statement validating historical truth.

Not only in the treatment of trauma survivors, but also in the treatment of all patients where the therapist and patient work only with material that is reported, the focus is on helping to resolve the patient's suffering and not on establishing historical accuracy.

Some other possibilities suggested for contamination of memory include persuasion by therapists, hypnotic suggestibility, recalling someone else's experiences as one's own memories, hysterical contagion as in the spread of rumors, mistaking fantasy for reality, deception, substituting a false memory for a more painful reality, confusing memory that was encoded during states of disorganization as a preverbal or immature child incapable of storing memory realistically, and others. Even in dissociative disorders, a variety of coexisting yet different realities are believed simultaneously.

There are a variety of explanations for false memory. Although these explanations have been hypothesized, many have not been studied. Further, there is a great deal of research information about memory that is learned from nonclinical populations that may not apply to you. Professionals have a lot to learn about memory processing in nontraumatic situations and about memory processing in survivors of abuse. One cannot necessarily translate information about memory in nontraumatized people to those who were traumatized. It is hoped that the issue of false memory and the polarized viewpoints among professionals can be put aside so that you can receive the best possible treatment for your condition.

You also need to know that many people have been successfully treated and feel better after entering treatment for their traumatic and dissociative conditions. Although treatment approaches may continue to change as professionals learn more, we feel that treatment results do provide a significant hope and expectation for improvement so that you can enter treatment with an understanding that many people have markedly improved or recovered.

I have read the above information about the treatment of my condition. I have discussed questions I may have had and understand the complexities involved in my treatment and with memory in general. I understand I can assist in my treatment planning and I can discontinue treatment at any time. I agree to treatment based on my own informed wish to proceed and at my own risk as well as my potential benefit.

Patient's signature   Date

Witness   Date

Informed Consent for Use of Clinical Hypnosis

Before deciding to participate in clinical hypnosis, it is important that you understand how clinical hypnosis is used in treating dissociative and traumatic disorders. Hypnosis is a valuable tool but has been the subject of considerable controversy among clinicians in the field. For this reason, it is important that you understand some basic issues about hypnosis to be adequately informed.

Hypnosis is an altered state of consciousness that has a number of characteristics. These include a capacity for deep absorption in the hypnotic state with a reduced awareness of external events, an altered perception of one's reality, a high level of suggestibility, and a suspension of critical judgment, including evaluating information retrieved during the hypnotic state. These characteristics are more prominent in people who have dissociative conditions, and therefore more contaminations of memory and information retrieved in hypnotic states occur. All of these features combine to increase the possibility of producing inaccurate, distorted, or false memories. The hypnotic state can result in confusion among reality, one's fantasy life, suggestions or demands from a therapist, and influence of other stimuli occurring in hypnosis that may alter the realistic interpretation of retrieved information.

Research on hypnosis has demonstrated that hypnosis may enhance memory but also may distort or lead to the production of false information that is perceived as memory. This is due to the nature of hypnosis, the demand quality inherent in some hypnotic suggestions, and the individual's expectations of what a therapist may want to discover. Further, information may be retrieved in a hypnotic state that is accompanied by high levels of intensity, body sensations, and a conviction that the information is accurate, despite evidence that the information was the product of contamination or hypnotic suggestion. On the other hand, hypnosis is capable of enhancing real memory and retrieving real information that has been repressed or forgotten. Individuals in a hypnotic state may not be able to distinguish the difference between information that is accurate and information that is artifact.

The accuracy of hypnotic retrieval of dissociated memory for traumatic events has not been adequately studied. The uncertainty of hypnotic memory retrieval means that information retrieved in hypnosis should be accepted only with caution and a recognition that it may or may not be historically correct. There is no way of knowing whether any information that is retrieved through hypnosis is historically accurate. Historical accuracy can be determined only by the independent validation of information that is retrieved. This is true of all memories reported in psychotherapy. These issues are particularly relevant for individuals with dissociative conditions because they are often highly suggestible and therefore prone to the complications of hypnosis in which suggestibility, suspension of critical judgment, and absorption in the experience may allow even greater degrees of distortion.

People with dissociative disorders are prone to accepting suggestions whether they are placed in formal hypnosis or not. Dissociative individuals are often in states of autohypnosis or self-induced trance, especially during psychotherapy sessions or periods of stress.

There are other sources of contamination. Subjects retrieving memories in hypnosis may recall information heard from other sources, or even may recall their own fears or fantasies, and experience them as though they were memories. Individuals forget the original source of the information and subsequently feel as though it originated in themselves, attributing the emerging material to memory. This phenomenon, known as *source amnesia*, is well known in hypnosis and can be very compelling.

Beyond the issue of memory, it is exceedingly important to be aware that in many legal jurisdictions and in different states the use of hypnosis may have an impact in litigation. Experiencing hypnotically refreshed memory, for example, or simply undergoing hypnosis may prevent or disqualify individuals from testifying in legal proceedings. It is important that you be aware of this in the event that you are involved in a legal action or expect that you might use information that you learn in your treatment in a future legal action. Hypnosis may impede or prevent you from testifying. You may want to contact your attorney if the potential for litigation is relevant.

There are other complications that may occur with the use of hypnosis. These include flooding of emotions, flashbacks, traumatic imagery, and highly charged traumatic memories, leading to increased disorganization, suicidality, and self-destructive or aggressive behaviors. Hypnosis might result in premature emergence of information that you do not feel ready to manage. These problems may occur and produce the same symptoms without clinical hypnosis.

Hypnosis, on the other hand, has many potential values. It may be used effectively for reducing anxiety, developing internal states of relaxation, or inducing guided imagery that can help during periods of crisis. Hypnosis also may help gain information that is unavailable because it is contained in dissociated states. It also may be valuable in developing an internal dialogue between, or an awareness of, other internal states.

Hypnosis is not required for your treatment, and many people have successfully completed treatment without it. You can participate in traditional forms of psychotherapy, groups, and cognitive and behavioral techniques, and you can use medications and emotional containment strategies to develop a sense of safety in your treatment.

I have been fully informed about the pitfalls and potential advantages of hypnosis. I am also aware that other forms of treatment, such as psychotherapy, group therapies, cognitive therapies, and others, are used very successfully and may reduce some of the risks surrounding memory distortion. I understand and give my consent to the utilization of hypnosis, knowing that I may discontinue at any time.

Patient's signature   Date

Therapist   Date

CHAPTER 5

Satanic Ritual Abuse: First Research and Therapeutic Implications

Philip M. Coons, M.D.

*B*eginning in the early 1980s, reports of child abuse involving satanic rituals began to circulate, primarily among clinicians dealing with child abuse and severe dissociative disorders (Blood 1989; California Office of Criminal Justice Planning 1989–1990; Los Angeles County Commission for Women 1989; Nurcombe and Unützer 1991; Smith and Pazder 1980). These rituals were alleged to occur within the context of a "vast international, multigenerational conspiracy" (Putnam 1991). Bizarre rituals of torture, human and animal sacrifice, perverted sex, sexual and physical abuse, cannibalism, necrophilia, and breeding of babies for human sacrifice were described by both adults and children. These rituals were reported to occur in basements of homes, churches, and day care centers and to involve black-robed persons using satanic paraphernalia such as candles, altars, knives, and other satanic symbols. Children describing such rituals were participants in some of America's biggest day care–center trials (Pendergrast 1995). Adults describing satanic ritual abuse (SRA) usually had severe dissociative disorders, including dissociative identity disorder (DID; formerly called multiple personality disorder) and dissociative disorder not otherwise specified or DDNOS (Feldman 1993; Hill

105

and Goodwin 1989; Mulhern 1994; Ofshe 1992).

Clinicians reacted quickly to these horrible accounts of abuse, and soon professional books, articles, and workshops on how to recognize and treat victims of SRA proliferated. Television talk shows, often of a highly dramatic nature, were also produced, not to mention hundreds of newspaper and magazine accounts (Blood 1989). Soon controversy arose over the literal existence of SRA. Proponents of both positions took extreme stands either by wholeheartedly embracing the existence of SRA (Blood 1989; Los Angeles County Commission for Women 1989; Smith and Pazder 1980) or by denying its existence from an extremely skeptical viewpoint (Ofshe 1992; Pendergrast 1995; Richardson et al. 1991). Balanced professional reviews of the SRA literature are hard to find, with one exception (Rogers 1992). Despite extensive law enforcement investigation throughout the United States, no good corroborative evidence of SRA has ever been found (Lanning 1992).

In the past few years, another intimately related phenomenon has arisen—the so-called false memory syndrome (FMS). Proponents of FMS have formed the False Memory Syndrome Foundation, headquartered in Philadelphia, Pennsylvania. Members consist mainly of parents who claim to have been falsely accused of child abuse, usually sexual, by their now-adult children, primarily daughters. The foundation's advisory board members consist of many luminaries in the field of memory research. Advocates of FMS allege that therapists iatrogenically create false memories through suggestion or even outright coercion. Accounts of retractors, or those patients who initially thought that their parents had abused them sexually but now believe that such abuse did not happen, have begun to emerge (Goldstein and Farmer 1993). Recently, reports of SRA have been postulated to be entirely a phenomenon of false memory (Pendergrast 1995).

The clinical and political climate has become increasingly polarized in the midst of accusations of abuse and vociferous denials (Gutheil 1993). One factor underlying this polarization has been the recent liberalization of statutes of limitations in many states allowing adult children to sue their parents for decades-old child abuse (Spiegel and Scheflin 1994). Recently, malpractice suits have been filed by parents alleging that their daughters' therapists have created false memories. At least one third-party suit filed against therapists by a parent has recently been successful (Grinfield and Duffy 1994). Polarization has become so great that several professional organizations have issued policy statements about the nature of memory and the recovery of repressed memories (American Medical Association 1994; American Psychiatric Association 1994; American Psychological Association, in press; British Psychological Society 1995; Canadian Psychiatric Association [Blackshaw et al. 1996]). Legislation has been proposed in the United States Congress and several state legislatures (Hirsh 1994) to regulate what has been labeled "repressed memory therapy" (Ofshe 1992; Ofshe and Singer 1994).

Unfortunately, although unsubstantiated opinion and belief about memory and repression in general and SRA in particular abound and often approach a religious fervor, research regarding repressed memory and reports of SRA has only recently begun. The literature on memory and repression is so vast that only a few review articles are cited for the interested reader (Brown 1995; Lindsay and Read 1994; Loftus 1993; Read and Lindsay 1994). However, recent research on forgotten memories of child abuse appears to indicate that repression is possible in a sizable minority of patients (Briere and Conte 1993; Feldman-Summers and Pope 1994; Loftus et al. 1994; Terr 1994; Williams 1994).

Research on Satanic Ritual Abuse

Interestingly, the first research on SRA was not performed by psychiatrists or psychologists but by sociologists and anthropologists (Balch and Gilliam 1991; Mulhern 1994; Richardson et al. 1991; Victor 1989, 1991). These scientists failed to find objective evidence that SRA literally occurs. Instead, they believe that SRA develops as a rumor or folk legend whose spread is fueled by media hype, Christian fundamentalism, mental health and law enforcement professionals, and child abuse advocates.

One example of a rumor panic about satanic cults occurred near Jamestown in western New York in May 1988 (Victor 1989, 1991), when school officials from numerous schools in the area reported hundreds of children absent because of parental fears of satanic abuse. There were reports of mutilated animals, satanic graffiti, and corpses being found. The police were deluged with telephone calls; town meetings were held, and prayer meetings were held in churches. Subsequently, from a search of small-town newspapers, Victor (1991) documented evidence of 61 other satanic cult rumors in widespread locations across the United States. These rumors occurred between 1982 and 1993 and peaked in 1988 and 1989. Unfortunately, it is impossible to tell from Victor's cursory review of the evidence what really did happen at these 61 locations. There is no question, however, that reports of satanic activity provoked a media frenzy in many locations.

In an interesting case report, Coons and Grier (1990) discovered an additional explanation for SRA reports. They reported on a young woman with Munchausen syndrome who traveled from hospital to hospital, falsely claiming that she was a victim of SRA. In a now classic paper, Ganaway (1989) hypothesized that SRA might have alternative explanations besides the literal truth. These alternative explanations included fantasy, hallucination, delusion, screen memory, suggestion, or hypnosis, which created an illusion or false belief of having been involved in SRA.

Young et al. (1991) reported 37 consecutive adult patients diagnosed with either DID or DDNOS who reported childhood SRA. These patients included 33 women and 4 men who were treated in four separate sites in the United States. Interestingly, many of the SRA reports developed while the patients were hospitalized in special dissociative disorder inpatient units where they had ample opportunity to interact with other dissociative disorder patients. It is also interesting to note that many of their experiences were strikingly similar and many had retrieved their memories under hypnosis. None of the cases was referred for law enforcement verification, and no collateral interviews were held with family members to verify the abuse because patients feared retaliation. Although evidence of previous physical injury was found on physical examination in some of the patients, these injuries could have been self-inflicted.

Jonker and Jonker-Bakker (1991), two family physicians, reported on SRA in Oude Pekela, a town of 8,000 in northern Holland. In 1987, a 4-year-old boy presented with anal bleeding with no clear physical cause. Over the next few days, he gave an account of sexual abuse and subsequently implicated 25 other children. During the next 18 months, a law enforcement investigation was launched, and there was a proliferation of publicity. In all, 98 children, ages 4–11 years, were implicated in what was described as SRA. Jonker and Jonker-Bakker conducted a questionnaire survey of the parents of 90 of the children and asked about any behavioral disturbance the children might have had during and after the alleged SRA and their own beliefs about the possibility of SRA. Of these parents, 87% were certain that their children had been involved in SRA. Although two suspects were temporarily detained by the police, they were released because of lack of evidence.

Recently, Coons (1994) did a retrospective review of psychiatric records of 29 patients who reported SRA during their evaluation in a dissociative disorders clinic. Of these patients, 76% had dissociative disorders, either DID or DDNOS. SRA stories were judged to be delusional in three cases and factitious in another four cases. No external corroboration of SRA was obtained in any of the cases, despite intense medical and legal investigation in about one-fourth of the cases, which were involved in civil malpractice litigation. Extensive law enforcement investigation in an additional three cases reported to the police also provided no confirming evidence. In fact, investigation in three cases produced evidence from the physical examination directly contradicting patients' accounts. These included two baby breeders, one of whom was a virgin and the other of whom had a nonparous cervix. The third patient alleged that the cults had carved satanic symbols on her back, but no scarring was found (Coons and Grier 1990). Many of the patients were thought to have confabulated memories of SRA through hypnotic memory retrieval, guided imagery, or group work. In other cases, patients and therapists were thought to have misinterpreted dream material as evidence for SRA. In only two patients were no questionable therapeutic practices found.

Two large studies of SRA reports are now completed but are not yet published (J. S. La Fontaine: "The Extent and Nature of Organized and Ritual Abuse: A Report to the Department of Health," 1994; G. S. Goodman, J. Qin, B. L. Bottoms, et al.: "Characteristics and Sources of Allegations of Ritualistic Child Abuse: Final Report to the National Center on Child Abuse and Neglect," 1995). The La Fontaine study was commissioned by the British government as an independent, non-law-enforcement study of allegations of ritual abuse (RA) of children in England and Wales. There were 79 reported cases of RA during a 4-year period from 1988 to 1991. The number of cases peaked at 29 in 1989, and there was only 1 reported case in 1992. La Fontaine had access to all of the police and social service records generated in each case and also interviewed key persons, including police, social workers, parents, and foster parents. None of the children were reinterviewed to avoid subjecting them to further trauma. None of the cases involved preschool-age children as has occurred in the United States. Material corroborative evidence was found in only three cases, two of which occurred in 1983. This evidence consisted of altars, candles, costumes, and photographs. None of these confirmed cases involved witchcraft or satanism but instead involved a single perpetrator who claimed spiritual powers. In 38 cases, verbatim interviews of the children were studied in detail and many revealed poorly conducted interviews, repeated at short intervals and including leading questions. In about 80% of the cases involving allegations of RA, no charges were ever brought because of lack of evidence. In addition, the RA cases had the lowest rate of conviction (21%) when charges were brought. There was no evidence that forced abortion, human sacrifice, cannibalism, or bestiality occurred in any of the cases. It appeared that the disclosures of RA by the younger children were greatly influenced by adult caregivers.

Goodman et al. investigated characteristics and allegations of SRA and religion-related abuse (i.e., clergy abuse or withholding medical care) in a series of five studies. In the first study, they surveyed psychiatrists, psychologists, and social workers who reported seeing a total of 1,061 cases of SRA. Although these clinicians were asked about corroborative evidence of intergenerational satanic cults that sexually abuse children, none was found. However, a few cases were found where lone individuals or, at most, two people abused children. Soft evidence, including scars, was reported, but they could have been self-inflicted. In addition, this study concluded that clinicians routinely believed the allegations of SRA.

In the second study, Goodman's group surveyed district attorneys, law enforcement agencies, and social service agencies for cases of SRA. Although physical evidence such as satanic graffiti, books, and artifacts was found, often there was little corroborative evidence that children had been abused or harmed. The third study focused on 43 repressed memory cases from the first study. In none of these cases was corroborative evidence found indicating the existence of the horrible SRA described at the beginning of this chapter. In the fourth study, Goodman's group examined children's knowledge of SRA (none of these children had been abused) and found that they did not have knowledge about satanic activity associated with sexual abuse. This finding led researchers to the conclusion that children were unlikely to invent stories of SRA by themselves. Finally, in the fifth study, when researchers compared religion-related abuse with SRA, they found more convincing corroborative evidence of religion-related abuse than of SRA.

Therapeutic Implications and Personal Reflections

A number of good references concerning guidelines on how to deal with repressed memories of previous child abuse have recently been published (American Psychiatric Association 1994; Bloom 1994; Brown 1995; Ganaway 1989; Lindsay and Read 1994; Lynn and Nash 1994; Watkins 1993; Yapko 1994). My purpose is not to repeat these guidelines in detail but to interpret them and describe how I deal with persons who report SRA.

An extremely thorough diagnostic evaluation is essential. This evaluation should include present and past psychiatric histories, medical history, social history, and mental status examination. If the patient describes physical evidence of abuse on his or her person, he or she should be referred for a physical examination. In particular, the examiner should carefully examine the skin and genital areas for evidence of abuse, and the clinician should remember that abuse can be self-inflicted. Remember also that if the patient alleges delivering babies for sacrifice, the cervix should be parous. If the patient refuses referral for physical examination, records of previous physical examinations can be obtained with the patient's permission. Likewise, previous psychiatric records should be obtained. Finally, collateral examination of family members may give clues about the patient's veracity. Thorough diagnostic evaluations enable the astute clinician to separate patients who have delusional beliefs about SRA, or those who have factitious disorders and are fabricating stories of SRA, from the remainder of the patients who report SRA.

Patients with psychoses or factitious disorders constitute a minority of patients who report SRA. Their treatment follows, in general, the treatment of the primary disorder; however, this treatment is not further described here. But what of the patients who report SRA and are not psychotic or factitious? How should they be treated? Many of these patients have severe dissociative disorders as primary diagnoses, and these disorders should be treated.

What follows is my general approach to dissociative disorder patients who report SRA. I have found that these patients are extremely sensitive and often question me about my belief in SRA, sometimes over the telephone before their first appointment. I try to remain neutral and indicate that because I was not present at the reported abuse I cannot make a judgment about its historical occurrence. Most importantly, I try to examine why my belief in SRA is so important to them.

I have found that memories of SRA have nearly always been repressed or forgotten and then remembered through a variety of mechanisms, including dreams, hypnosis, flashbacks, and guided imagery. I am very careful to educate these patients about the vagaries of memory and the nature of hypnosis and dreams (American Psychiatric Association 1994; American Medical Association 1994; American Society of Clinical Hypnosis 1995; British Psychological Society 1995; Brown 1995; Lindsay and Read 1994; Loftus 1993; Read and Lindsay 1994). Patients need to understand that memory is not like a tape recorder and that dreams are highly symbolic. Furthermore, hypnosis or Sodium Amytal does not ensure adequate recall.

I rarely use hypnosis or Sodium Amytal to explore memory, but when I do, I inform patients that what is retrieved may not be factual, that their belief in the factual nature of the material will be increased, and that any subsequent testimony about previous abuse in a court of law may be disallowed. I am extremely careful not to suggest abuse to patients, whether or not they are under hypnosis or Sodium Amytal.

Rarely can I or the patient quickly determine the factual nature of reported abuse. Sometimes we never can. Thus, we must both learn to tolerate uncertainty and ambiguity. I help the patient understand that the memory may either be literal or derive from a dream or a metaphor, or there may be elements of both. I try not to impose my beliefs or suspicions upon the patient. It is up to the patient to decide for himself or herself whether events really did happen.

Initially, my focus is on stabilizing the patient, and the patient's stability remains important throughout therapy. A patient's functional status is of paramount importance to me. I do not schedule abreactive sessions to work through trauma; rather, after patients are stabilized, traumatic memories are worked through gradually as they arise. Variants of this phase-specific treatment of posttraumatic memories have been described elsewhere (Herman 1992; Kluft 1993; van der Hart et al. 1993).

I neither encourage patients to confront their abusers or to file lawsuits against their abusers, nor will I agree to be a witness in such a lawsuit. My duty is to be a therapist to the patient. I cannot serve two masters by being both an expert witness and a therapist. If patients do wish to confront their abusers or file lawsuits against their abusers, I insist that they first consider all the consequences of doing so. So far, only 1 patient in more than 300 dissociative disorder patients has filed a lawsuit against her abuser, and she had always remembered her abuse. Although many patients wish to avoid family members who have abused them, I encourage them to keep other family relationships. I do not insist that they forgive their abusers.

As a final note, I must state that patients who report SRA and do not have evidence of either factitious disorder or psychosis truly believe that they were victims of SRA. Because these patients perceive that they suffered from SRA, they express real emotions, such as anger, horror, disgust, or depression. These feelings must be respected.

Conclusion

There currently is little objective evidence that accounts of SRA involving the horrific practices of breeding babies, human sacrifice, cannibalism, and intergenerational or international SRA conspiracies are literally true. Some patients who report SRA have either psychoses or factitious disorders. It is likely that there are alternative explanations to the literal truth in those who report SRA and do not have psychoses or factitious disorders. These alternative explanations include hypnotic confabulation and misinterpretation of dreams and fantasy. Treatment of individuals who report SRA should stress a thorough diagnostic evaluation, avoidance of suggestion, therapeutic neutrality, toleration of uncertainty and ambiguity, education, and respect for the patient's feelings and boundaries.

References

American Medical Association Council on Scientific Affairs: Memories of childhood sexual abuse (CSA Rep No 5-A-94). Chicago, IL, American Medical Association, 1994

American Psychiatric Association Board of Trustees: Statement on memories of sexual abuse. Int J Clin Exp Hypn 42:261–264, 1994

American Psychological Association: Working Group on Investigation of Memories of Childhood Abuse. Washington, DC, American Psychological Association (in press)

American Society of Clinical Hypnosis: Clinical Hypnosis and Memory: Guidelines for Clinicians and for Forensic Hypnosis. Chicago, IL, American Society of Clinical Hypnosis Press, 1995

Balch RW, Gilliam M: Devil worship in western Montana: a case study in rumor construction, in The Satanism Scare. Edited by Richardson JT, Best J, Bromley DG. New York, Aldine de Gruyter, 1991, pp 249–262

Blackshaw S, Chandarana P, Garneau Y, et al: Adult recovered memories of childhood sexual abuse (position paper, Canadian Psychiatric Association). Can J Psychiatry 5:305–306, 1996

Blood LO: Satanism and Satanism-Related Crime: A Resource Guide. Weston, MA, American Family Foundation, 1989

Bloom PB: Clinical guidelines in using hypnosis in uncovering memories of sexual abuse: a master class commentary. Int J Clin Exp Hypn 42:173–178, 1994

Briere J, Conte J: Self-reported amnesia for abuse in adults molested as children. J Trauma Stress 6:21–31, 1993

British Psychological Society Working Party: Recovered Memories. Leicester, England, British Psychological Society, 1995

Brown D: Pseudomemories: the standard of science and standard of care in trauma treatment. Am J Clin Hypn 37:1–24, 1995

California Office of Criminal Justice Planning: Occult Crime: A Law Enforcement Primer: Research Update 1(6). Sacramento, California Office of Criminal Justice Planning, 1989–1990

Coons PM: Reports of satanic ritual abuse: further implications about pseudomemories. Percept Mot Skills 78:1376–1378, 1994

Coons PM, Grier F: Factitious disorder (Munchausen type) involving allegations of satanic ritual abuse: a case report. Dissociation 3:177–178, 1990

Feldman GC: Lessons in Evil, Lessons From the Light: A True Story of Satanic Abuse and Spiritual Healing. New York, Crown Publishers, 1993

Feldman-Summers S, Pope KS: The experience of "forgetting" childhood abuse: a national survey of psychologists. J Consult Clin Psychol 62:636–639, 1994

Ganaway GK: Historical versus narrative truth: clarifying the role of endogenous trauma in the etiology of MPD and its variants. Dissociation 2:205–220, 1989

Goldstein E, Farmer K: Confabulations: Creating False Memories, Destroying Families. Boca Raton, FL, SIRS, 1993

Grinfield MJ, Duffy JF: Jury awards father $500,000 in recovered memories trial. Psychiatric Times, June 1994, pp 1, 7

Gutheil TG: True or false memories of sexual abuse: a forensic psychiatric review. Psychiatric Annals 23:527–531, 1993

Herman JL: Trauma and Recovery. New York, Basic Books, 1992

Hill S, Goodwin J: Satanism: similarities between patient accounts and pre-Inquisition historical sources. Dissociation 2:39–44, 1989

Hirsh KS: Legislating memory. MS Magazine, July–August, 1994, p 91

Jonker F, Jonker-Bakker P: Experiences with ritualistic child sexual abuse: a case study from the Netherlands. Child Abuse Negl 15:191–196, 1991

Kluft RP: The initial stages of psychotherapy in the treatment of multiple personality disorder patients. Dissociation 6:145–161, 1993

Lanning KV: A law enforcement perspective on allegations of ritual abuse, in Out of Darkness: Exploring Satanism and Ritual Abuse. Edited by Sakheim DK, Devine SE. New York, Lexington Books, 1992, pp 109–144

Lindsay DS, Read JD: Psychotherapy and memories of childhood sexual abuse: a cognitive perspective. Applied Cognitive Psychology 8:281–338, 1994

Loftus EF: The reality of repressed memories. Am Psychol 45:518–537, 1993

Loftus EF, Polonsy S, Fillilove MT: Memories of childhood sexual abuse: remembering and repressing. Psychology of Women Quarterly 18:67–84, 1994

Los Angeles County Commission for Women: Report of the Ritual Abuse Task Force: Los Angeles, CA, Los Angeles County Commission for Women, 1989

Lynn SJ, Nash MR: Truth in memory: ramifications for psychotherapy and hypnotherapy. Am J Clin Hypn 36:194–208, 1994

Mulhern S: Satanism, ritual abuse, and multiple personality disorder: a sociohistorical perspective. Int J Clin Exp Hypn 42:265–288, 1994

Nurcombe B, Unützer J: The ritual abuse of children: clinical features and diagnostic reasoning. J Am Acad Child Adolesc Psychiatry 30:272–276, 1991

Ofshe RJ: Inadvertent hypnosis during interrogation: false confession due to dissociative state, misidentified multiple personality, and the satanic cult hypothesis. Int J Clin Exp Hypn 40:125–156, 1992

Ofshe RJ, Singer MT: Recovered memory therapy and robust repression: influence and pseudomemories. Int J Clin Exp Hypn 42:391–410, 1994

Pendergrast M: Victims of Memory: Incest Accusations and Shattered Lives. Hinesburg, VT, Upper Access, 1995

Putnam FW: The satanic ritual abuse controversy. Child Abuse Negl 15:175–179, 1991

Read JD, Lindsay DS: Moving toward a middle ground on the "false memory debate": reply to commentaries on Lindsay and Read. Applied Cognitive Psychology 8:407–435, 1994

Richardson JT, Best J, Bromley DG (eds): The Satanism Scare. New York, Aldine de Gruyter, 1991

Rogers ML (ed): Special issue: satanic ritual abuse: the current state of knowledge. Journal of Psychology and Theology 20:175–339, 1992

Smith M, Pazder L: Michelle Remembers. New York, Pocket Books, 1980

Spiegel D, Scheflin AW: Dissociated or fabricated? psychiatric aspects of repressed memory in criminal and civil cases. Int J Clin Exp Hypn 42:411–432, 1994

Terr LC: Unchained Memories: True Stories of Traumatic Memories: Lost and Found. New York, Basic Books, 1994 van der Hart O, Steele K, Boon S, et al: The treatment of traumatic memories: synthesis, realization, and integration. Dissociation 6:162–180, 1993

Victor JS: A rumor panic about a dangerous satanic cult in western New York. New York Folklore 15:23–49, 1989

Victor JS: The dynamics of rumor-panics about satanic cults, in The Satanism Scare. Edited by Richardson JT, Best J, Bromley DG. New York, Aldine de Gruyter, 1991, pp 221–236

Watkins JG: Dealing with the problem of "false memory" in clinic and court. Journal of Psychiatry and the Law 21:297–317, 1993

Williams LM: Recall of childhood trauma: a prospective study of women's memories of child sexual abuse. J Consult Clin Psychol 62:1167–1176, 1994

Yapko MD: Suggestions of Abuse: True and False Memories of Childhood Sexual Traumas. New York, Simon & Schuster, 1994

Young WC, Sachs RG, Braun BG, et al: Parents reporting ritual abuse in childhood: a clinical syndrome: report of 37 cases. Child Abuse Negl 15:181–189, 1991

CHAPTER 6

Ritual Abuse:
Lessons Learned as a Therapist

George A. Fraser, M.D., F.R.C.P.C.

*O*ver the past 8 years, in dealing with patients recalling ritual abuse (RA), I have had to do much soul searching as well as literature searching to comprehend what I was being told by this very distressed group of patients. After having been involved in the treatment of more than 40 such patients, I have as yet been unable to sort out fully, to my own satisfaction, exactly what has led to this phenomenon. I doubt anyone has the full answer. I have, however, learned many lessons in the course of my clinical work. This phenomenon has caused me to be more cautious in uncritically accepting abuse memories. On the other hand, there have been disturbing considerations that cannot be discounted and have left me with the uncomfortable feeling that within this maze of satanic confusion lies the possibility of truth in some patients' reports.

This chapter then is not an argument for or against the reality of RA but rather a sharing of my clinical experiences and dilemmas in working in this field. I divide this chapter into three sections:

1. Lessons learned that have led me to be cautious in accepting what I am told by patients
2. Factors that lead me to accept the possibility of RA
3. Changes in my approach to new patients presenting with RA histories, resulting from the previous two factors

In central and eastern Canada, I was one of the first therapists to begin hearing reports of RA. This is probably not surprising because I had already partially specialized in managing multiple personality disorder (MPD), now called dissociative identity disorder (DID; American Psychiatric Association 1994). RA recollections occur mainly in this group of MPD/DID patients. Previously, I had read only a few papers and attended a couple of seminars on RA. RA was not a phenomenon I ever expected to see in Canada.

Soon after, when patients in my practice began reporting RA memories, I was concerned about managing them in relative professional isolation because of my lack of clinical experience with this patient group. I was hearing about horrendous sadistic abuses, murders and burials, and cults that were reportedly operating in secrecy. I began to feel rather uneasy about working with RA patients. I wondered if I had a civic responsibility to report these alleged unknown murders to the police. Could the patients be in danger for telling me? Might I be delving into an area I may very soon regret? What of safety for my staff? What of my family's safety? To the best of my knowledge, none of my colleagues in Ottawa were hearing these stories. However, I knew colleagues in other centers who had encountered patients with similar histories. I telephoned some therapists who had experience in this area. I also contacted the Ottawa Police Force. To my relief, the police worked in cooperation with me and my initial RA patients for almost a year.

Other therapists who began treating patients with RA memories have had similar experiences as mine. Relating my experiences, I hope, may better prepare therapists encountering the RA phenomenon for the first time to deal with similar issues. For those who deride RA, I hope this chapter will help them understand the difficulties encountered by therapists who have tried to comprehend this complex issue while managing these patients. RA continues to be a difficult subject because therapists have to balance the possibility of reality with that of hysteria, malingering, or errors in memory recall. It is easier to sit in the comfort of a chair at home and judge as a philosopher than to sit in the office with a patient revealing memories of RA. Conversely, it is easier to overreact in the therapist's chair. Continued dialogue from those representing both sides of the RA issue will one day help to establish the true center of balance. I do not believe we have found that point yet, but we are getting closer.

Lessons Leading to Skepticism of Patients' Histories

Lacking the Body of Evidence

The police, who interviewed a number of my patients having recollections of RA, had visited sites with a few MPD/DID patients where they believed ceremonies or burials had taken place. No evidence was ever uncovered to support these claims. This lack of evidence also was noted by Lanning (1989), of the U.S. Federal Bureau of Investigation (FBI). Eventually, the police said that without evidence other than memory recollections in this group of patients, there was nothing to be gained by searching areas for proof. This viewpoint of the police made my life as a therapist much easier. Without evidence other than memories, I no longer felt a need to contact the police. These patients, of course, were free to report their memories to the authorities if they wished, but I would advise them first of my collaborative experience with the police.

Credibility Problem

The police were concerned about the credibility of some of my patients. For example, one 19-year-old patient reported an abduction and rape by her uncle and another man whom she had known from the cult. The abduction and rape were said to have taken place the previous evening, after the patient left her cousin earlier that same evening. The police had already been working with this patient, and I felt that because the event was so recent, we might be able to prove her allegations. I asked her if she had gone to the hospital for a medical examination after the rape. She said she was so angry with her last hospital experience after having been raped that she had not gone. Nonetheless, this assault was recent, so with her permission I called the police, who quickly established that she was not raped that evening—her cousin had been with her that entire evening. The patient then changed her story and said that the rape had actually happened the day before. She said she lied because she thought rapes had to be reported within 24 hours to be investigated. Although the police were somewhat frustrated, to their credit they decided to continue to follow up on the lead of this other male (the uncle had a valid alibi) because the patient was sure she knew him and where he lived. Having followed all their leads, the police concluded that no such person existed. This report was only one of a number of unreliable reports this patient gave. She did it so often that in my mind she became the girl who cried wolf. I knew that if anything did happen to her in the future, I would have problems seeking cooperation from the police because she had totally destroyed her credibility in their eyes. This credibility issue was a problem the police noted in other cases they investigated. One police investigator summarized the year's work by saying, "Possibly a third of what we were told might have happened, one-third was lies, and the other third likely was merely fantasy."

Source Amnesia

Another patient presented an alter personality who related a very detailed abuse episode that had an uncanny ring of familiarity. It suddenly dawned on me that this was an abuse story written in *Michelle Remembers* (Smith and Pazder 1980). Her story was so much like the book that I am almost positive this was not the experience of this patient. The alter personality had other recollections as well that led me to doubt the authenticity of the patient's story. I do not believe the patient intended to lie. She had a host of books about satanic cults that I had earlier asked her to stop reading. I believe that when she read *Michelle Remembers,* this alter began to believe that Michelle's abuses were her own experience. In time, the likely source of the event, the book, was forgotten. Such a phenomenon has been called *source amnesia.*

Factitious Disorder

A young woman with an atypical dissociative disorder told of difficulties separating reality from her fantasies. She told of a report she made to the police relating an abduction and rape. She went to the hospital for examination and gave details to the police of the attacker and the color of the car he had used. The police launched an investigation, but the attacker was not found. The problem was that the event did not occur. She later admitted to me that she had missed work and made up this rape story as an excuse. But what began as malingering became more complicated and more like a factitious disorder. By the time the police were involved, she was firmly convinced the rape had indeed happened. I asked if I could videotape her recollection of the entire scenario to use for teaching psychiatric residents how a fantasy can change to reality for some highly hypnotizable people (she had a 10/10 hypnotic induction score) (Spiegel and Spiegel 1978). Halfway through the videotaping, she paused and said in fact she now believed the rape had occurred. I told her I could not help her because I had no idea of the facts. Shortly thereafter, she seemed to regain her conviction that it did not happen. The rape probably did not happen, but the experience revealed that this patient had honest difficulties separating fact from fantasy.

I believe that factitious disorder (Munchausen syndrome) is probably more common than has been previously suspected. More study is needed in the area of malingering, factitious disorder, and reports of RA. I suspect factitious disorder patients may at times believe their own stories, as in the case previously described, whereas in malingering, patients knowingly lie.

Grade 5 Syndrome and the Fantasy-Prone Personality

If hypnotic trance state potential is measured, there is a group who have the ability to enter very deep trance levels. These virtuosos of trance states have what is called Grade 5 syndrome, as measured by the hypnotic induction profile (HIP; Spiegel and Spiegel 1978). Such individuals not only score at the top of the HIP, but also "are usually capable of experiencing age regression in the present tense, sustained post-hypnotic motor alterations and hallucinatory responses in compliance with a cue, and/or global amnesia for the entire hypnotic episode. If the individual is capable of all of these experiences, he is considered a grade 5" (Spiegel and Spiegel 1978, p. 317). Spiegel and Spiegel estimated about 5% of the population fit into the category.

Although I did not go beyond the HIP to test for Grade 5 syndrome, a fair number of patients over the course of therapy exhibited these specific phenomena, indicating they would fit into this grouping.

There appears to be some overlap with the Grade 5 syndrome group and another group, who frequently are also hypnotic virtuosos, independently described (Wilson and Barber 1982). Wilson and Barber used the term *fantasy-prone personality* (FPP). They estimated that 4% of the population may be so hypnotizable that they have trance experiences that, to them, are as real as real. They may have hallucinations in all sensory modalities and can have difficulties separating fantasy from reality. Memories of fantasies can appear as real as real. Wilson and Barber compared a group with FPP with a control group and outlined the various hypnotic phenomena experienced in the virtuoso group. I have had MPD/DID patients with recollections of RA who can fit into one or both of these groups. I believe we now have to look more closely at Grade 5 syndrome and FPP concepts and determine how extreme hypnotic capacity and FPP can impair a person's ability to separate fantasy from reality. Grade 5 syndrome and FPP may explain the origin of some memories that patients attribute to RA and possibly some reports of abductions by unidentified flying objects (UFOs).

In my own practice, I have encountered Grade 5 syndrome and FPP among my MPD/DID and RA patients. One patient who fits the criteria for both Grade 5 syndrome and FPP told me, "The difference between you and me is that when you fantasize, you know it's fantasy. Often, I can't tell the difference. I've had to learn that fantasy is part of my reality." Grade 5 syndrome and FPP concepts must be understood by all therapists dealing with RA and MPD/DID.

Recently, I spoke to a middle-aged male patient who fits the criteria for both Grade 5 syndrome and FPP. He told me that one of his fondest childhood memories had been going to Disneyland with his parents and a friend. Even now, he can recall the smells and taste of the candy. He also can recall the noise of the rides and the many colors of the theme park. He even recalls the feeling of being on the rides. The problem is that he only recently found out from his mother that he was never there. She reminded him of his abusive alcoholic father who never took the family anywhere, let alone Disneyland. He now realizes this was a fantasy he had created. The child who shared the rides with him was his imaginary childhood companion.

He is not the only patient who has informed me that inner trance experiences can be as real as outer reality. As clinicians, we must remember that a certain number of our patients may be relating trance experiences and fantasies that in fact did not happen anywhere else but in their minds. These trance experiences and fantasies may well be possible explanations for some RA reports; patients are not lying but instead have a fantasy memory.

Sabotaging Alters

A patient stated that she had been warned by her cult to stop seeing me, but she ignored these warnings. Soon, she began getting "blackmail letters" as she called them. She was distressed and said this was the beginning of her end because she had not heeded the warnings to stop seeing me. She showed me a few of these letters. They consisted of a black envelope addressed to her in white lettering. Each was from a different country, and the stamps bore what appeared to be the appropriate cancellation postmarks. One letter was from Hong Kong, one was from the USA, and yet another was from Portugal. Each letter contained two tarot cards, one of the devil, the other of death. She said this would continue on a regular basis until she received the seventh black letter, which would be from Switzerland. The letter from Switzerland would contain a third tarot card indicating the way she was to commit suicide for breaking the secrecy.

Later, she phoned my office and said the seventh black letter had arrived from Switzerland. She was afraid to open it. I rather dramatically told her not to open it but bring it to my office immediately. I confirmed the stamp and postmark date and opened the letter. The extra tarot card depicted a hanging scene. I refused her requests to let her see the card (I feel somewhat naive as I recount this story). I turned the envelopes over to the police. The result: the letters were all forgeries. Because of the black envelope, it was easy to have the cancellation postmark of the stamp appear to blend in.

The source of the letters were other alters who were trying to frighten the patient. As I look back, there was a certain element of *la belle indifference* in her reaction to the seventh letter. When I told her the police's conclusion that the letters were forgeries, the topic was immediately dropped and she never discussed it again.

This same patient had been frightened by the delivery of a package that contained a dead bird. She believed this was a warning from her cult. She now knows it was the work of one of her cultic alter personalities. I later learned that when the police were investigating some of my other patients who had received warning signs, such as satanic markings on the sidewalks outside their homes, these were observed to have been done by the patients themselves. After fusion or integration, a patient admitted that the ominous markings that had terrified her had been done by one of her alter personalities, although she stated that she herself was not aware of this at the time. She said the alter had done it to discredit her for telling the RA stories.

From these cases I learned that threats of danger to myself, although infrequent, may well have originated from alter personalities of my patients. If therapists feel they have been threatened, I suggest they consider an alter personality as the source of the problem. However, I do not intend to suggest that all threats and warnings can be attributed to inner cultic personalities. Nonetheless, a threatening alter is not to be ignored. I do know of therapists who have been assaulted by alter personalities. I advise my patients that aggression of any type toward me by either them or an alter would likely lead to termination of therapy.

Staged Events

Patients have repeatedly told stories of being administered drugs during ceremonies. These reports alerted therapists to the possibility that recalled memories could include the recall of drug-induced hallucinations. We also must consider that highly hypnotizable persons who are in a heightened state of suggestibility are capable of being tricked. The following case illustrates this phenomenon:

> A patient was most upset as she recalled giving birth to a cult baby within the cult and having to participate in the murder of that infant. She recalls being given an injection. After she worked on

the memory of that event, I asked if she would review that memory as though she were watching it as a passive observer. She immediately commented, as she reviewed the memory in this manner, that she had not in fact been pregnant. She reported being led through a simulated delivery by those around her. An alter personality had been led to believe she was pregnant. At some stage, a small animal was produced, which she was told was her own newly delivered baby. It was this animal that was supposedly killed.

At the end of the session, the patient felt convinced that this had been a staged event in which she had been tricked into believing that she was pregnant and had delivered and killed her own child.

Of course, I have no way of knowing the truth of any of these events, but certainly this patient, who no longer dissociates, is convinced she was the victim of a planned false memory. This case does not indicate that all of my patients who have recollections of infanticide are merely reporting false memories.

Other patients told how they, as children, were hidden in various locations during cult ceremonies to operate special effects and to set up optical illusions to fool cult initiates into believing supernatural events were happening. If this is true, then cult participants, including our patients, at times may have been exposed to cleverly staged theatrical events that were misinterpreted as being of supernatural demonic origin.

These examples, which are not unique to my experience, point out the difficulties that confront the therapist who assists patients with recollections of RA. There are many ways to distort recalled memories; however, this does not mean that hypnosis and other methods cannot help in recalling accurate memories. True recollection under hypnosis does occur (American Medical Association 1985), but therapists must be aware that such recollections do not always lead to the truth. At this point, I doubt anyone can honestly claim always to know when a recalled memory is true, false, or only partly true.

Although staged events demonstrate that what is recalled by patients may not be fact, the phenomenon of sadistic abuses cannot be discounted simply as false memories or hysteria.

Factors Leading Me to Believe
Reports of Ritual Abuse Could Be True

Patients Reporting Ritual Abuse

The most obvious factor leading me to consider the possible reality of RA cults is that there are patients reporting these cult abuses. For many, the conviction of abuse by a cult remains unshaken even after integration and therapy. Because some recalled memories in non-RA cases have been true, we are obliged as therapists to at least consider that some RA memories could be true.

The paradigm from which many of us view life does not include the types of cruel abuses heard about in satanic cults. We should remember Shakespeare's advice as spoken by Hamlet: "There are more things in heaven and earth, Horatio, than are dreamt of in your philosophy." Perversions and sexual tortures are a reality in our society, and some victims eventually end up in the mental health system. Perhaps the stories are fantasies, perhaps lies, but also perhaps they are the truth. We must deal with all possibilities rather than profess we know the answer without evaluating each case on its own merits.

Contaminating the Victim's Credibility

Long before I had encountered RA or MPD/DID or knew anything about hypnosis, I had an interesting experience as a medical doctor in the Canadian Armed Forces. A private was sent to me who claimed he was tied to a tree and sodomized by his platoon sergeant. He had reported this assault to his commanding officer the previous evening. He stated he and the sergeant were in the woods to witness a diamond smuggling ring between Barbados and Toronto via this military base. He said gunshots had been fired and that two bodies were floating in the nearby river. It was during this melee that he had been tied and sodomized. The Royal Canadian Mounted Police were called, but no bodies were found in the river. The sergeant indignantly denied the whole affair, and everyone agreed the private's story was just too far-fetched to be believed. The young private was referred to the provincial psychiatric hospital, although he never did change his story during the months he spent as an inpatient. About 6 months later, two events happened on the same day. The doctor across the hall consulted me to help diagnose a patient with an unusual type of hemorrhoids. I walked into his office where the patient was still bent over exposing the supposed hemorrhoids. I recognized the problem immediately as a large perianal wart (condyloma acuminatum). I had previously treated this condition on the accused sergeant's penis. As can happen sometimes in small communities, another coincidence had happened: earlier, I also had diagnosed vaginal condylomata acuminata on the accused sergeant's wife while assisting the civilian doctor in the nearby community. The patient in my colleague's office then pulled up his pants and turned around. It was the very same private who had claimed he was sodomized. Condylomata acuminata can be sexually transmitted. This diagnosis seemed to support the private's sodomy story. I was considering my legal responsibility and to whom I should report this information, but that same morning the military police called me and told me that the sergeant and his wife were under arrest. Schoolchildren in the community alleged that they had been sexually abused by the sergeant and his wife. The two confessed to all the reports of abuse, including sodomy by the sergeant on the young private. The sergeant's modus apparatus was to destroy the credibility of the victim in advance. In the case of the private, it was to tell the victim a ridiculous story (diamond smuggling), and later, after luring him into the woods under the pretext of witnessing the smuggling, the sergeant fired some shots in the air and convinced the private that people had been killed. The sergeant then carried out the sexual abuse knowing that if the private reported the abuse he would not be believed because the entire set of events was too incredible and without evidence. The sodomy really did happen, but he was tricked into also believing the other events that did not happen. The sergeant's plan worked, and the innocent private had spent useless months as a psychiatric inpatient. Neither his military unit nor the psychiatric staff, nor myself, had believed him. A few days after the sergeant's arrest, there was a tap at my office door. The young private stuck his head inside the room and slowly said, "I told you so, sir!" then he left with a satisfied grin on his face. That experience stayed with me and has left me more cautious about discounting events when they seem incredible or improbable. Could some of our patients' stories of the satanic ceremonies be a cover-up for the real issue—sexual abuse? The lesson here is that false beliefs can be induced to discredit true memories. Both could be present at the same time; it is not necessarily an either-or situation.

Silence of the Group

It has been argued that sexual abuses in groups could not continue for years without anyone finding out. Therefore, satanic ritual abuse could not have gone undetected in our current media-aware culture where communications are at a very advanced state.

A number of recent incidents in Canada have been uncovered contradicting this theory. Two major scandals stand out: one in Newfoundland and the other in my home province of Ontario. In both, sexual abuses on a relatively large scale had gone undetected for years.

The nation was shocked when it was revealed that several Christian Brothers at Mount Cashel Orphanage in Newfoundland had sexually and physically abused boys for years. Abuses by the clergy had occurred there and in other locations for almost 20 years before the reports of victims were taken seriously (Archdiocese of St. John's 1990).

The scandal in Ontario involves a boys' training school run by Christian Brothers in the town of Alfred. This case became public knowledge in 1990. Sexual and physical abuses had gone on for 30 years. There are more than 150 former male students claiming abuse while they were students. There have been convictions, and financial compensation for the victims has been arranged. A colleague who had been practicing in the area recently confided to me that about two decades ago he had assessed two boys from that training school who had told him they were being sexually abused. He said he did not believe them at the time and assumed they had made up these allegations to get away from the reform school. No action was taken. In retrospect, he regrets his cynicism. Such was the attitude of the time.

Finally, it might be argued that these two events occurred in institutions, unlike a satanic cult, which would operate within a community. This argument can be laid to rest with the uncovering of a widespread community-based sexual abuse scandal that took place a mere hour's drive from my hospital. In that community, during a period of 25 years, there were numerous sexual abuses in group settings involving children and adults. On March 25, 1995, the *Ottawa Citizen* reported that 275 children had been molested (178 female and 97 male) and that of 122 suspected child abusers, 65 had been charged, 52 trials were completed (with a conviction rate of 90%), and 12 trials are pending. The case remains ongoing. Although there were initial reports suggesting satanic rituals, the case was handled solely as an abuse issue without the satanic reports being addressed. This case does prove that widespread sexual abuse can exist secretly within a community. Although rumors were heard sporadically in all three cases, they were considered too incredible to be believed and the abuses continued.

Common Alleged Abusers

In a previous article, I referred to two patients who had identified common abusers (Fraser 1990). At the time, neither patient had met the other for years nor knew I was treating the other (one had moved to Ottawa from outside the province, and the other had to fly to Ottawa for therapy sessions from a different location). Because neither had spoken of the other in therapy and because both patients mentioned three identical abusers, I wondered if they were connected in common abuses. Confidentiality did not allow me to discuss one patient with the other. Eventually, the link became evident. A relative of one of these patients had been a housemate of the other patient. That relative had frequently been identified by both as an abuser within what each called a satanic cult. Other common abuse locations had been discussed independently. Eventually, the patients did meet and recognize each other and found out I was treating them both, but they did not talk to each other until they requested a meeting in my office with me present. They spoke of similar abusers whom each patient had mentioned to me previously and described an abuse scene in which both were involved. Although I admit their account of RA is not independently verifiable, it nonetheless is an event that has stayed in my mind. Although I am more cautious and skeptical than I was when I wrote that article in 1990, I am still not able to discount the stories of those two patients.

It is too facile and too premature simply to discount all reports of abuses in ritualized settings merely because some can be explained by false recollections.

Current Approaches to Patients Reporting Ritual Abuse

All of the previously described lessons have led me to be cautious about believing and disbelieving the phenomenon of sadistic or satanic cults and reports of RA. They also have influenced how I approach new cases today.

My current approach to patients who have memories of RA is as follows:

- I advise the patient that therapy can be very stressful and lengthy, and it is not to be undertaken lightly.
- I state there is no guarantee that recalled memories are necessarily accurate or true, even if they are elicited by hypnosis or Sodium Amytal (also referred to colloquially as "truth serum").
- When asked by patients if I believe their recollections of RA, I answer that I *believe* that these abuses could have happened, but without corroboration, I cannot *know* they happened.
- I am no longer overly concerned about safety for myself and my staff, provided we maintain our normal professional boundaries with RA patients. I remind patients that safety in therapy must be respected by them as well as myself.
- I do not try to prove whether cults do or do not exist. I do not call the police when ritual murders are mentioned; however, I suggest the patient may do so if he or she wishes or feels there is concrete evidence. Naturally, if I believe there is concrete evidence, I treat this like any other case where a known murder is involved.
- I remind myself that I am a therapist, not a detective.
- I accept that false memories can occur. I also accept that true

memories can occur. I remind the patient that although recalled memories can be true, there is also the possibility of false or distorted memories.

- I remind the patient that hypnotic recall of memories could interfere with his or her ability to use recalled material in future court cases (American Society of Clinical Hypnosis 1995).
- If a patient states that he or she continues to be harassed, I suggest that the patient consider the possibility of alter personality sabotage. If sabotage by an alter is not the case, he or she has the right to contact the police and seek a restraining order if an external harasser is known.
- I remind psychiatric residents and others whom I may lecture to avoid asking the patient leading questions. We must listen, then question, but not suggest.
- If patients fear the process of uncovering memories, I remind them that resistance is a form of protection. Sometimes it is better to go slowly or not at all rather than force abreactions or memory recall before a patient is ready. Forcing patients to delve into memories too soon can be unnecessarily stressful. If the patient's current life is going well, it may be appropriate to avoid uncovering past amnesic periods.
- Finally, because of my experience with the media while treating RA patients, I am reluctant to talk to the media unless they review with me any quotes or statements they wish to publish. Often they will refuse. Too often, reporters concentrate on the satanic aspect of RA stories and seem to lose focus of what was actually said. It is probably better that patients avoid the media because once patients recover, they may regret being videotaped and seeing the recording rerun for the public. If an answer to the media is important, then I would consider the policy of one chief executive officer. He asks the media source to write, fax, or E-mail questions and he replies in writing, which minimizes the times the media might misrepresent sources.

Conclusion

I have addressed issues of RA using examples from my own caseload. Because patients have reported dramatic and frightening stories, as well as criminal activities, therapists are ensnared in perhaps the most controversial issue in psychiatry since Sigmund Freud abandoned his theory of childhood seduction as a cause for adult hysteria and proposed the fantasy hypothesis, in which he stated that most adult reports of childhood seduction had never occurred (Jones 1953). As therapists, we are caught between the cries of patients recalling horrific memories of abuse and the cries of colleagues proclaiming "satanic panic."

Currently, the facts of the RA phenomenon are not yet known. I have offered examples from my experiences suggesting there are factors that contribute to patients' erroneous histories. I also have explained why I and other therapists have concerns that at least some histories of cult RA could be based on actual events. Patients cannot be abandoned by simply calling their memories "fantasies."

References

American Medical Association Council on Scientific Affairs: Council report: scientific status of refreshing recollection by the use of hypnosis. JAMA 253:1918–1923, 1985

American Psychiatric Association: Diagnostic and Statistical Manual of Mental Disorders, 4th Edition. Washington, DC, American Psychiatric Association, 1994

American Society of Clinical Hypnosis Committee on Hypnosis and Memory: Clinical Hypnosis and Memory: Guidelines for Clinicians and for Forensic Hypnosis. Des Plaines, IL, American Society of Clinical Hypnosis, 1995

Archdiocese of St. John's: The Report of the Archdiocese Committee of Enquiry into the Sexual Abuse of Children by Members of the Clergy, Vol 1, 1., 1. Newfoundland, Canada, Archdiocese of St. John's, 1990

Fraser GA: Satanic ritual abuse: a cause of multiple personality disorder. Journal of Child and Youth Care (Special Issue):55–65, 1990

Jones E: The Life and Work of Sigmund Freud, Vol 1. New York, Basic Books, 1953

Lanning K: Satanic, occultic ritualistic crime: a law enforcement perspective. The Police Chief 56 (10):62–83, 1989

Smith M, Pazder L: Michelle Remembers. New York, Pocket Books, 1980

Spiegel H, Spiegel D: Trance and Treatment: Clinical Issues of Hypnosis. New York, Basic Books, 1978

Wilson SC, Barber TX: The fantasy-prone personality: implications for understanding imagery, hypnosis and parapsychological phenomena, in Imagery: Current Theory, Research, and Application. Edited by Sheikh A. New York, Wiley, 1982, pp 340–347

CHAPTER 7

Ritual Abuse in European Countries: A Clinician's Perspective

Onno van der Hart, Ph.D.
Suzette Boon, Ph.D.
Olga Heijtmajer Jansen, M.D.

*T*here is a growing concern among Dutch clinicians treating patients with multiple personality disorder (MPD), now called dissociative identity disorder (DID; American Psychiatric Association 1994), in the phenomenon of satanic ritual abuse (SRA) and its psychological sequelae for survivors of such an extreme form of abuse (satanic cult survivors or SCSs). At the same time, an increasing number of Dutch child therapists working in residential settings are considering DID and SRA in children in whom other forms of child abuse are already proven. Different police agencies across the country have been faced with cases of children and adults reporting SRA. In recent years, a much larger number of SRA cases involving children also has been reported in Great Britain.

SRA is receiving considerable attention in North America and is the subject of intense debate, particularly among law enforcement officers and clinicians treating MPD/DID patients (Ganaway 1989; Hill and Goodwin 1989; Kahaner 1988; Lanning 1991; Putnam 1991; Van Benschoten 1990; Young et al. 1991). Therefore, a report on SRA in Great Britain and the Netherlands may be of special interest to North American readers.

The Los Angeles County Commission for Women (1989) defined ritual abuse as follows:

> A brutal form of abuse of children, adolescents, and adults, consisting of physical, sexual, and psychological abuse, and involving the use of rituals. Ritual does not necessarily mean satanic. However, most survivors state that they were ritually abused as part of satanic worship for the purpose of indoctrinating them into satanic beliefs and practices. Ritual abuse rarely consists of a single episode. It usually involves repeated abuse over an extended period of time.

In this chapter, we adhere to the commission's definition. However, because all reported or alleged ritual abuse cases mentioned within this chapter refer to satanic practices, we use the term *satanic ritual abuse*. Greaves (1992) distinguished four positions interested professionals may take regarding SRA and SCSs: 1) nihilist, 2) apologist, 3) heuristic, and 4) methodologist. Nihilists seem to explain away the allegations of SCSs (i.e., their reports cannot be true). Apologists seem to explain why the reports of SCSs must be true. Heuristics are mainly a large group of clinicians who are uncommitted to any objective conclusions about the whole matter but who have found that treating their SCS patients' reports in a confirming manner has resulted in favorable outcomes in treatment. The methodological perspective, finally, is the least developed aspect of the SCS field. This perspective is further explored by Dr. Philip M. Coons in Chapter 5.

Our own position is as follows. In the past 10 years we have treated, as well as consulted other colleagues who have treated, adult patients whose reports or allegations of SRA seemed to be very convincing. The possibility of these reports or allegations being truthful had to be seriously considered because other explanations, such as "pathological distortion in order to get attention or sympathy," "distorted reality as resulting of (other) traumatic memories," "contagion by the media, therapist or others" (Lanning 1992), provided insufficient or no understanding of the very consistent symptoms and behaviors—allegedly related to SRA—of these patients. Several Dutch child therapists working in residential treatment settings reported equally convincing cases. However, we also believe that some reports of alleged SRA reflect the clinician's bias or the patient's tendency toward mythomania (Ellenberger 1970). We have observed a few patients whose reports of SRA were not convincing and very different from all other cases that we consider genuine. In these patients whose reports were not convincing, a severe personality disorder and a pathological distortion of reality in order to receive attention and sympathy seemed to be the most apt explanations for these allegations of SRA. Perhaps the best position is described by Van Benschoten (1990), who proposed that "an attitude of critical judgement concerning satanic ritual abuse is necessary, to avoid either denying the issue or overgeneralizing the nature and extent of the problem" (p. 22).

In this chapter, we present an overview of relevant material pertaining to SRA cases involving children in both Great Britain and the Netherlands, diagnostic issues regarding alleged SRA in children and adult DID patients in the Netherlands, treatment issues, and issues related to the credibility of SRA accounts.

Cases of Satanic Ritual Abuse Involving Children in Europe

Great Britain

In Europe, Great Britain is the country wherein most reports on SRA of children are being made. The National Society for the Prevention of Cruelty to Children (NSPCC) is alarmed about the increasing number of cases coming to its attention. Towns and areas mentioned are Hull, Surrey, Wolverhampton, Telford, Portsmouth, Manchester, and Shrewsbury, among others (Bartlett 1989; Tate 1991). Reports of SRA are typically made by social workers involved in ordinary child abuse cases or by foster parents of child victims of sexual and physical abuse. Within the context of an enduring relationship with an adult whom these children trust, the children disclose information that to a trained observer points to possible SRA. Typically, children's reports include adults carrying candles, wearing robes and masks or dressing up as clowns, and chanting;

children being defecated on, forced to eat body wastes, locked in cages or boxes, or sexually abused on crosses or inside stars and circles; drinking blood; sacrificing animals; torturing, killing, and consuming babies; being filmed by cameras with lights on; using drugs; and adults threatening children in order to discourage disclosure. Tate (1991), who examined a number of these British cases and compared them with North American and Dutch cases (Hudson 1991; Jonker and Jonker-Bakker 1991; Snow and Sorenson 1990), was struck by the similarities. Because many of these children reported SRA without attending adults encouraging them, Tate concluded that either there exists a worldwide conspiracy by toddlers or the children are speaking the truth.

The Nottingham case.   One of the most widely reported cases of SRA in Great Britain is the Nottingham case (Cohen 1990; Dawson and Johnston 1989; Tate 1991). After earlier reports on child abuse and neglect, it was discovered in 1985 that a few children from an extended family in Broxtowe, Nottingham, had been sexually abused by relatives. In 1987, 23 children from the family were sent to children's institutions and later to foster families. Ten adult members were arrested. Apart from showing the usual signs of sexual abuse, these children were extremely frightened and anxious. When feeling safer, they told their foster parents detailed information, including the torture and killing of babies, which was subsequently interpreted by the judge of this case as suggesting SRA. The social workers involved became convinced that this was a probable SRA case. The children's stories were confirmed by independent reports from three female members of the family who were not arrested. They also admitted having taken part, albeit under duress, in SRA, not only within their own extended family, but also during more grotesque rituals in the homes of rich, apparently wealthy (just as the children reported). However, the police agency on the case did not believe SRA existed and instructed the three female witnesses to keep completely silent on this issue. Therefore, in 1989 the 10 arrested family members were sentenced together to serve more than 150 years in prison because of incest, abuse, sodomy, and neglect. SRA, however, was not mentioned in the verdict as per instructions of the police agency.

In the meantime, the social workers involved heard more details of SRA and were against discarding evidence on this matter. They started their own investigation and found, for example, that the children's report on the existence of a tunnel used in the SRA, a report previously dismissed by the police, was true—a reason for even more animosity between the social workers and the police. Pressed by police, the new director of social services forbade social workers, in the summer of 1989, to talk about SRA in public. An inquiry team comprising two social workers and two police officers was established to determine whether satanism had been involved. The team released a careless report condemning the children's evidence as unreliable. However, social workers who believed that SRA was involved made their own report. In November 1990, the director of social services officially concluded that ritual abuse during satanic ceremonies was indeed likely to have taken place in Nottingham (Tate 1991).

Influenced by the Nottingham case, as well as by the increasing number of other reports of SRA, which the NSPCC continues to receive, the British government announced in March 1991 that it would support a 2-year study on the subject.

The Netherlands

Until 1993, little attention had been given in the Netherlands to the phenomenon of SRA. Before 1993, brief newspaper reports regarding SRA in countries such as Spain and Mexico and reviews of books such as *Cults That Kill* (Kahaner 1988) and *The Satanism Scare* (Richardson et al. 1991) appeared, and some special attention had been given to the Nottingham case in Great Britain.

On television, a Christian fundamentalist station broadcast three documentaries on SRA in the United States, alleging that similar phenomena were taking place in the Netherlands. Because of this station's religious orientation, these rather subjective programs were not taken very seriously by the public.

In 1986, a case of large-scale child abuse was reported in the city of Haarlem, in the western Netherlands, and became known as the Leidse Buurt Affair. Because the children involved reported filming of the abuse, allegations of child pornography were made.

Subsequently, clinicians treating some of these children became more knowledgeable about SRA and recognized signs of possible SRA in the verbal reports and drawings of these children. In recent years, more cases of child and adult SCSs have been discovered in the Haarlem region. The Leidse Buurt Affair is largely forgotten by the general public.

However, another case, with some similarities to the Nottingham case, shook the country in 1987.

The Oude Pekela case.   For years, the small town of Oude Pekela, located in the northern Netherlands, became the focus of attention of the mass media, the general public, police agencies, mental health professionals, and many self-proclaimed experts on mass hysteria.

A 4-year-old boy with anal bleeding presented to a general practice office in Oude Pekela during May 1987 (Jonker and Jonker-Bakker 1991, 1992a, 1992b). The initial evaluation revealed no clear cause for the anal bleeding. During the next few days, the child told a story of sexual abuse, including a history of sticks being inserted into his anus, and mentioned a friend who also had been involved. Both sets of parents collaborated and subsequently contacted the police. When the 4-year-old boy was medically examined again because of persistent anal bleeding, the mother told the attending physician about his story of sexual abuse and her contact with the police.

Law enforcement interviews began immediately. The two boys implicated 25 other children, who were subsequently interviewed. The total investigation time lasted 18 months but did not produce any incriminating evidence such as admissions by offenders, photographs, or videotapes, although children reported being involved in filming activities. During this time, 98 children, ages 4–11 years, were interviewed. There was no possibility of all the children knowing one another because they lived in different areas and attended different schools. Younger children (ages 3–6 years) were implicated early, but eventually cases of older victims became known. Usable information was provided by 62 of the children, and 48 children gave clear statements of sexual victimization. The children told of events consistent with large-scale ritualistic abuse, the essence of which follows (Tate 1991):

... being abused by a large number of adults who chanted in a strange language; sometimes the adults dressed as clowns, other times as lions and bears. The children claimed that these mysterious adults walked around the children in a circular dance, tied them up or locked them in cages; they forced the children to eat faeces and drink urine or blood. Drugs were administered and babies mutilated or killed. Cameras had captured much of this on film or video. (p. 235)

Differences of opinion among physicians, criminal investigators, and the public prosecutor developed. The Justice Department invited a child psychiatrist, Dr. Gerrit Mik, to determine whether something had actually happened to the children. Mik heard, and saw in the children's drawings, many bizarre details, which he could not place initially. He then found that these children's stories and drawings contained elements very similar to those reported by child SCSs in the Nottingham case. Then, the bizarre information provided by the children of Oude Pekela began to make sense.

In the meantime, however, authorities did not inform parents of the progress of the investigation, which infuriated the parents. In January 1988, an anonymous group of parents wrote a letter outlining their children's experiences and distributed it throughout the community. The entire town experienced a severe crisis, the mass media plagued the town, and the general public was upset.

Self-proclaimed experts publicly expressed their opinion that the whole affair could be reduced to a simple case of mass hysteria, based solely on the play between two boys who pricked each other in the anus with a little stick (e.g., Rossen 1991, 1992). Because there were no arrests or charges, a large portion of the general public, including many mental health professionals, accepted this version. However, Tate (1991) reported that the police privately admitted that at least 32 children had been abused and that another 25 were likely to have been victims. According to Tate, police did not admit that the abuse had taken place during rituals, as the children alleged, or as part of an organized ring of pedophiles.

In 1995, Karel Pyck, a Belgian professor of child psychiatry, published the results of his in-depth study of the Oude Pekela case. He concluded that the abuse reports were essentially true. There was no evidence whatsoever that the case was merely a product of mass hysteria. Pyck attacked Rossen, the originator of the mass hysteria hypothesis, for his extreme bias and his very selective use of available sources.

Other Developments

In 1992, 11 allegations of SRA of children were made to the Inspection for Youth Mental Health and the Justice Department. This information was eventually shared with the authoritative news program "Nova," on national television, which in June 1993 dedicated a series of two programs to the subject of SRA. Representatives of police departments and the Justice Department, as well as therapists and victims, presented their views on the matter. The foundation Korrelatie, a public agency that people may call for emotional support following emotionally charged television programs and other events, subsequently received 112 telephone calls; 35 callers reported ritual abuse. Subsequently, questions were raised in Dutch Parliament, and the justice minister ordered the formation of a task force to investigate further the subject of ritual abuse. Members of this task force spoke with alleged victims, clinicians of child and adult survivors of SRA, and police representatives. In April 1994, the task force presented its report, with the major conclusion that no forensic evidence for the existence of ritual abuse had been found. Therefore, the validity of allegations of ritual abuse/SRA did not seem to be likely. However, the task force also concluded that the lack of forensic evidence did not necessarily mean that all reports of ritual abuse/SRA were baseless. The task force recommended further investigation and the formation of an organization to which clinicians could report cases of (alleged) ritual abuse/SRA, which would allow for a more systematic investigation. These recommendations have apparently not been followed through. Clinicians who in 1993 publicly spoke about SRA as reported by their patients now keep such information to themselves. Not reporting information is partially the result of the false memory debate regarding the validity of "recovered memories" of childhood sexual abuse, in which false memory proponents use allegations of SRA as an argument to invalidate the phenomenon of recovered memories (e.g., Crombach and Merckelbach 1996).

In September 1996, SRA again received media attention. A Dutch commercial television channel dedicated a series of six programs to SRA and DID. None of the clinicians participating in the 1993 television programs agreed to participate. Police officers mentioned that since the appearance of the above mentioned task force report, very few reports of SRA have come to their attention. We have the impression, however, that in cases of sadistic sexual abuse involving organized perpetrators, both public prosecutors and police officers overlook the satanic aspects of reported abuse, focusing instead on the ordinary criminal aspects such as pornography, drug dealing, and child kidnapping for sexual abuse.

An example is the Den Helder case. In early 1996, the parents of a 12-year-old girl from Den Helder, a town in the northern Netherlands, were convicted, along with other adults, of sexually abusing the child over a period of time. Although expert witnesses concluded that the victim's reports of sexual abuse were valid, they thought her allegations about rituals in which, among other things, animals and human beings were killed were less valid. However, there is no proof that the assumptions of the expert witnesses are factual, yet their conclusions can be misinterpreted to mean that SRA was *not* involved.

Following the first four of these television programs, the foundation Korrelatie reported 16 telephone calls in which ritual abuse was mentioned. Twelve callers stated that they were victims of SRA, and four mentioned that a family member or friend is, or has been, involved in a satanic cult. The majority of 81 callers expressed anger at individuals who in these programs stated their doubt or disbelief about the validity of SRA and of the dissociative disorders. Korrelatie mentioned that the telephone conversations with the 12 alleged victims of SRA were characterized by fear and terror.

Satanic Ritual Abuse and Dissociative Identity Disorder: Diagnostic Aspects

North American therapists usually identify adult SCSs when treating patients who have DID. Generally, these patients first report other forms of abuse and eventually, hesitantly, disclose SRA.

Outside the Netherlands, DID is not widely diagnosed and treated as such in Europe. For instance, in Great Britain, most psychiatrists and psychologists still seem to believe that DID is a North American culture-bound phenomenon that is extremely rare in this country (Aldridge-Morris 1989; Fahy 1990). Because DID is rarely recognized as such in Great Britain, it is less likely that British therapists would detect signs of possible SRA in these patients. Nevertheless, the number of diagnosed DID patients is increasing in Great Britain (Karle 1992; Macilwain 1992; van der Hart 1993), and in some cases SRA is mentioned. The same is true in several other European countries, particularly Belgium and Germany (Huber 1995; van der Hart 1993). The first in-depth German study of a DID patient with a background of severe home abuse, child prostitution, and SRA has been published (Fröhling 1996).

Children With Dissociative Identity Disorder Reporting Satanic Ritual Abuse

Although many European therapists have not diagnosed and treated adult DID patients, a number of social workers in Great Britain involved in treating child SCSs have diagnosed DID in some of these children (Tate 1991). In the Netherlands, too, a few therapists of institutionalized child SCSs have diagnosed some of them as having DID (van der Hart and Boon 1991). These children had been placed by child protection services in residential treatment settings because of severe sexual and physical abuse and neglect. Physical and psychological evidence of their abuse was found by specialist physicians and psychologists. Because SRA was unfamiliar to them, these specialists were unaware of the meaning of the signs and symptoms suggesting SRA. The children alleged SRA only during the course of individual therapy within these institutions. Drawings depicting SRA themes are common, but therapists initially did not recognize these as a possible sign of SRA. For example, one drawing by a 5-year-old girl showed 1) a box with an inverted cross and the number 666 on it, with two people in the box described as "a mister above a little child"; 2) another figure with horns on his head, the number 666 on his body, and a knifelike object in each hand, with an inverted cross below this figure; 3) a table with an inverted cross and the number 666; on the table, a baby covered with blood; at the other side of the table, slightly above the baby, a figure depicted as "the boss," with an ax in one hand, horns on his head, the number 666 on his body, and an inverted cross below it; 4) a figure called "daddy"; 5) the figure of a child described as the patient's sister; and 6) a figure denoting the patient. One is again reminded of Tate's ironic suggestion that a worldwide conspiracy of toddlers exists.

In general, therapists treating child SCSs believed that the children had to feel safe with an adult with whom they had an enduring relationship, such as their individual play therapist, before talking more openly about SRA. This observation also was made in the Nottingham case; child SCSs told their stories only to individuals whom they felt they could trust (e.g., foster parents) (Tate 1991). They also described the threats they had received for disclosing SRA (e.g., their siblings or mother would be killed should they ever talk about SRA).

A recurrent observation in the Dutch institutions was that child SCSs who were visited in the institution by family members allegedly involved in a perpetrator organization, or, even worse, who occasionally went home for a weekend, invariably became highly symptomatic after the visits. They showed sexually provocative behavior toward other children and were more anxious, aggressive, reticent, and absentminded; they felt very insecure; and they complained of nightmares, headaches, or other physical symptoms. Typically, these children began to wet their beds again, refused to return to therapy, and showed marked distrust of adult caregivers and therapists. In addition, the children became aversive to disclosing more information. When some degree of trust eventually was reestablished, it was found that they had been threatened not to talk about the abuse.

The fact that these child SCSs also had MPD/DID was not discovered easily. Therapists observed over time that MPD/DID most aptly explained not only the extreme mood and behavioral variations in these children, but also the amnesic episodes that they showed.

Case Example

Daan was admitted to the institution at age 5 years because of severe sexual and physical abuse, his father and an uncle being the perpetrators, and emotional and pedagogic neglect (van der Hart and Boon 1991). During one of the first play-therapy sessions, he took a baby doll and a knight with a big knife. Although Daan tried to hide it, the play therapist observed that he let the knight put the knife in the baby. During some sessions, he was rather cooperative, but at other times he refused to enter the playroom. Then he became very angry and aggressive, shouted abuses at the therapist, and threw tables and chairs throughout the room. This pattern of destructive behavior had started when the therapist, who at the time was unaware of SRA, had arranged drawing paper and pencils for him. In a sudden attack of rage, Daan threw these materials around the room. Curiously, soon after such a sudden rage attack, Daan would go happily to the therapist and ask when he could come again to play, leading the therapist to suspect amnesia.

With time, Daan provided some information on SRA, and the therapist only began to recognize SRA when she contacted the therapist of Daan's mother, who independently had received similar information from the mother and had identified it as pertaining to SRA. It also became clear that Daan was systematically intimidated not to relate anything about SRA or else his mother would be killed. When this issue was resolved, Daan was able to relate his SRA experiences in play therapy. To do so, he had to first cover himself briefly with a blanket. When he reappeared, he seemed changed—older and wiser—and he talked more slowly, more detached, and more adultlike. During this treatment stage, Daan's therapist recognized and established contact with three alter personalities. She subsequently met with more alters, among them introjects of key figures of the perpetrator organization (independently identified as such by Daan's mother).

Adults With Dissociative Identity Disorder Reporting Satanic Ritual Abuse

Since the first workshop on DID in the Netherlands in 1984, given by Dr. Bennett Braun of Chicago, a steadily growing number of

Dutch clinicians from all over the country have been diagnosing and treating DID patients (Boon and Draijer 1991, 1993a, 1993b; van der Hart and Boon 1990).

The subject of SRA was first introduced to a few Dutch clinicians when Dr. Braun asked them during the 1984 workshop if they knew about SRA in the Netherlands or any other European country. They were completely unfamiliar with the subject. During the following years, more workshops were given on diagnosis and treatment of DID, and Dutch clinicians consulted American colleagues on certain severe symptoms and behaviors of some extremely complex DID patients. These clinicians were then informed that the severe symptoms and behaviors might possibly be related to experiences of SRA. By 1988, at least four DID patients had in the course of their treatment reported SRA experiences (van der Hart and Boon 1990). Since then, more Dutch clinicians, who had become familiar with signs and symptoms of SRA, reported treating DID patients who had alleged SRA.

Boon and Draijer (1993a) described the clinical phenomena of 71 Dutch DID patients. Follow-up data on this cohort of patients indicate that 38.8% of the patients ($N = 27$) had reported some form of SRA in the course of treatment. These patients lived in different regions in the Netherlands and they were treated by 19 different clinicians (Boon and Draijer 1993b). In this study, spontaneously given accounts of ritual abuse and drawings on the subject showed a striking resemblance to those of North American patients (see also Young et al. 1991).

Clinical Picture of Dissociative Identity Disorder Patients Reporting Satanic Ritual Abuse

Most DID patients alleging SRA present a consistent set of severe symptoms over time. These symptoms include severe posttraumatic stress symptoms, somatoform symptoms, extreme unusual fears and phobias, and recurrent dissociative states during which they exhibit behaviors associated with traumatic experiences and during which they report SRA, substance abuse, recurrent self-mutilation such as cutting and burning, recurrent suicidality or feelings that one has to die, extreme feelings of guilt and shame, and indoctrinated belief systems. Typically, these patients had a long history of medical and psychiatric care, and these symptoms and behaviors were present before specific DID treatments were started.

Some clinicians became aware of a pattern of symptoms, including extreme anxiety, eating problems, and specific somatic complaints, manifested during specific days of the year. They then recognized that those days coincided with ceremonial dates on the satanic calendar. In other cases, the patients showed drawings or other materials—sometimes long before treatment had started—that concretely depicted traumatic SRA memories (Shaffer and Cozolino 1992; Young et al. 1991). One Dutch patient presented drawings made when she was age 4 years, showing satanic symbols and representing the sacrifice of babies. She took the drawings from her mother, who had kept all her childhood artwork. Another SRA patient told her therapist that she remembered an elementary-school teacher had warned her parents because she was drawing cemeteries all the time. The host personality of another DID patient brought albums to therapy with photographs of signs and symbols used in satanic cult rituals and other symbolic representations of cult rituals; the patient could not remember drawing these pictures. Then, after having given the therapist three drawings—one representing the devil, the second a target, and the third a star—she killed herself. The therapist had no idea that SRA was involved, and the issue was not discussed in therapy. It was only after the patient's death that the therapist became informed of SRA. If one takes the phenomenon of SRA seriously, then it makes sense to hypothesize that, by presenting the photographs, some alters of this patient had wanted to communicate about the SRA. Her subsequent suicide then can be understood as most likely having been caused by a self-destructive program.

In patients reporting or alleging SRA, the system of alter personalities is more complex than in other DID patients. In most cases, these systems of alter personalities are layered. The basic subsystem consists of alter personalities that are involved in the patient's daily life and that keep memories of home abuse. Most of these alter personalities are unaware of SRA experiences and express disbelief when confronted with reports or allegations from other alters of SRA. These alters apparently belong to different subsystems of personalities. They usually present narrative fragments of SRA during the course of therapy. There exists one-way amnesia between these different subsystems, with the "daily" alter personalities absent when alters with SRA experiences take over executive control, and not the other way around.

In some patients, the structure of alter systems is highly complex, with different types of subsystems allegedly created by perpetrator organizations using mind control techniques. These subsystems (or specific alters) are reportedly trained to perform specific criminal activities. These patients appear to be strikingly similar to those described by North American clinicians (e.g., Hammond 1992).

Reported or Alleged Types of Abuse

In DID patients with an alleged SRA background, different subsystems of alter personalities report four different types of abuse.

1. *Sexual, physical, and emotional abuse taking place in the home environment.* Usually, one or both parents are reported to be involved, often along with other perpetrators. In some of the child victims, the sexual abuse has been corroborated, and the perpetrators have been convicted.
2. *Ritual abuse associated with satanic worship.* All patients report participation in rituals that include chants, symbols, robes, and special languages used by leaders of the ceremonies. Rituals usually take place according to a satanic calendar. Common elements reported or alleged are sexual abuse of children and adults; witnessing of, or participating in, torturing and killing of animals, children, or adults; physical abuse; forced impregnation and sacrifice of one's own child (or fetus); forced cannibalism; forced drug usage; and being buried alive in coffins. While reporting such extreme experiences, alter personalities are usually extremely anxious, hardly able to relate such material without starting to reexperience them. They sometimes relate this material in drawings and often in mirror writing (i.e., writing backward). All patients refer to extreme intimida-

tions and threats to keep silent. Control is enforced by threatening that important others will be tortured or killed if they do talk, by creating drug dependency in some alter personalities, or by forcing the victim to become a perpetrator who thus can be blackmailed.

3. *Pornography and prostitution.* Most patients (i.e., specific alters in these patients) report being both victim and perpetrator in the production of pornography, or being exploited as prostitutes, apparently for financial benefit of a perpetrator organization.

4. *Mind control.* All patients report having been subjected to some form of mind control, basically to ensure their loyalty to the perpetrator group or organization. Some patients, in particular those with multilayered subsystems of alter personalities, appear to have been subjected to extremely sophisticated mind control techniques, including a combination of drugs and hypnosis, pain, terror, electric shocks, isolation, and sensory deprivation or sensory overstimulation. Similar reports are given in the North American literature (Gould and Cozolino 1992; Shaffer and Cozolino 1992; Young 1992; Young et al. 1991). Dutch patients report that the perpetrators involved with the mind control were often English- or German-speaking persons. Some of the perpetrators were known to the patients, but others were not. Patients allegedly subjected to these mind control programs display subsystems of alter personalities that are highly indoctrinated, and some seem narcissistically involved in serving the goals of the perpetrator organization. Such alter personalities believe that they are the chosen ones prepared for a new future organization (with worldwide power) in which they will participate. However, they seem to have been exploited for criminal purposes such as kidnapping children for child-sex rings and producing pornography and snuff movies both in the Netherlands and in other countries.

Profile of Perpetrator Organizations

The patients seem to indicate that they have been abused by different groups. All report that at least one parent or family member was part of the group. All patients report some degree of organization; sometimes a high degree of organization and funding has been reported. Some of these groups are alleged to have international connections. Several patients exhibit systems of alter personalities reporting, in different languages (particularly Dutch, German, English, and South African), SRA and other types of abuse. They report being abused in ceremonies in different countries such as Belgium, Germany, Italy, Norway, Spain, South Africa, Switzerland, the United Kingdom, and the United States. Some patients report having been in many different countries, not only for SRA ceremonies but also for the purpose of criminal activities such as those described in the preceding discussion of alleged types of abuse.

In recent years, Dutch clinicians increasingly have gotten the impression that many of these so-called SRA groups are linked with syndicated child-sex rings (Lanning 1992) and other forms of organized crime. SRA activities seem to be a screen—evoking disbelief among law enforcement agencies and other parties when reported—as well as a means to ensure loyalty in victims, which is accomplished by instilling terror and guilt.

Treatment Issues

Treatment of Child Dissociative Identity Disorder Patients Reporting Satanic Ritual Abuse

In the Netherlands, treating child SCSs with DID in residential treatment settings, as practiced by a few child therapists, is in its infancy. Therapists are in the process of familiarizing themselves with DID and SRA and are learning appropriate treatment approaches. A most important issue is that these children are at risk for being visited by some of their abusers or for being sent home. The validity of SRA is often not accepted by the child protection services because of skepticism and a lack of legal evidence. Consequently, these children are going home for weekends and vacations, and they are not safeguarded against an extremely abusive environment. When the children return to the residential treatment center after such home visits, they appear extremely frightened and increasingly symptomatic. It depends upon the individual judge in juvenile court whether or not children will be protected from their abusers and for how long.

Possible child SCSs are usually identified in inpatient treatment settings that offer only short-term stays. Children reporting SRA are judged to be too severely disturbed for placement in a foster family. However, no institutions offer the necessary long-term inpatient treatment for these children. The dilemma that therapists of child SCSs face is whether or not to treat DID and SRA. Because in most cases therapists cannot protect the children from their abusers and cannot provide appropriate long-term inpatient treatment, there is a pervasive feeling of discouragement. Fortunately, there are some cases in which the children's safety has been ensured and where treatment is gradually progressing.

Treatment of Adult Dissociative Identity Disorder Patients Reporting Satanic Ritual Abuse

Treatment of adult DID patients reporting SRA experiences follows the general stages of appropriate treatment for DID and other trauma-induced disorders (Boon and van der Hart 1995): 1) stabilization and symptom reduction, 2) treatment of traumatic memories, and 3) integration and rehabilitation. Although there was initially an optimistic stance regarding treatment prognosis of DID, clinicians gradually realized that therapy aiming at complete personality integration, including the treatment of traumatic memories, is not always feasible (Groenendijk and van der Hart 1995; Horevitz and Loewenstein 1994).

Horevitz and Loewenstein (1994) describe a category of DID patients who tend to remain in abusive relationships. They have a poor therapeutic prognosis and can be treated most effectively when therapy is geared toward symptom stabilization and crisis management rather than toward the integration of alter personalities and treatment of traumatic memories. Many DID patients reporting SRA seem to belong to this category that Horevitz and Loewenstein describe. Kluft (1994) reported that patients with a background of ritual abuse appear to progress "quite unevenly and unpredictably over the short run and about half as rapidly as patients who have never made such allegations" (p. 67). Dutch clinicians, too, report that treatment of such patients is arduous and protracted. Treatment of these SRA cases is complicated by at least two issues: safety and complexity of DID.

Safety. Safety is always a crucial issue in treating adult and child DID patients. In cases where there is ongoing abuse, the only focus of the treatment should be to help patients stop the abuse. Dutch clinicians have found that most of the adult DID patients reporting SRA and other abuses in the course of their treatment unfortunately appeared to continue to be abused by a perpetrator organization. We observed in a few cases that a prolonged episode in a psychiatric hospital had enabled patients to end the abusive relationships.

Unfortunately, when DID patients enter treatment, it is often not clear whether some kind of abuse is still going on. One reason for this obscurity can be that the alter personality (or the "daily system" of alter personalities) presenting in therapy may be unaware of ongoing perpetrator contact. According to clinical observations, those patients who at the beginning of therapy presented total amnesia for any trauma history eventually appeared to have very complex histories of trauma and were often abused by organized rings of perpetrators. Therefore, in working with those patients, we have learned to be very cautious.

Complexity. DID patients reporting SRA in the course of treatment appear to have more complex systems of personalities than other DID patients. They also differ from other DID patients because of the indoctrinated belief systems that may hamper therapeutic progression. Patients indicating that they have been subjected to intensive mind control appear to have the most complex structured layers of alter personalities. For these patients, it also seems to be extremely difficult to stop their tendency to stay in contact with the perpetrators.

When patients do succeed in breaking off contact with the perpetrators and when their dissociative barriers are dissolving, they tend to have intense feelings of guilt, shame, and suicidality related to "perpetrator behaviors" that they themselves have been forced to manifest. These issues are extremely hard to deal with in therapy.

In the Netherlands and elsewhere (Huber 1995), therapists treating DID patients reporting SRA are confronted with intense positive and negative transference and countertransference issues. Particularly hard to deal with is the issue of patients being both victims and perpetrators of abuse. Sometimes, therapists are confronted with extremely difficult ethical dilemmas, for instance, in cases where patients allege to participate in SRA of their own children or others' children. In the Netherlands, clinicians are not obliged by Dutch law to report the abuse. They can report, anonymously or not, to a "Vertrouwensarts," a regional Dutch agency consisting of physicians and social workers who investigate cases of child abuse. So far, credibility issues regarding alleged SRA often have prevented child protection services to take these cases seriously. Nevertheless, awareness among some of these agencies, as well as of the Inspection for Youth Mental Health, has been increased, only to be invalidated by the aforementioned report on ritual abuse by the Justice Department's task force.

For only a few of these SRA cases, treatment can be evaluated over the long term in an inpatient setting. Some patients were able to stop the contact with the perpetrator organization, and they continued outpatient therapy with an emphasis on stage 2 of treatment, the assimilation and integration of traumatic memories. In other cases, patients were discharged from a clinical setting after reaching some degree of stabilization. No attempts were made to treat traumatic memories of SRA or of any other kind of abuse because these patients lacked the ego strength to do so. Outpatient therapy continued to focus on stabilization.

In outpatient treatment settings, therapies for a majority of patients reporting SRA are supportive because of the complexity of the problems encountered.

Credibility Issues

Dutch therapists of suspected SCSs with DID are confronted with the SRA controversy, which seems to be more prominently discussed in meetings and other situations (e.g., requesting hospitalization for SRA patients) than is identified in publications. Because the SRA phenomenon is so extreme, disbelief of alleged SRA is easily understood. In the literature, cases of both child and adult SRA increasingly have been reported (e.g., Finkelhor et al. 1988; Fröhling

1996; Gould 1987; Gould and Cozolino 1992; Hollingsworth 1986; Huber 1995; Jonker and Jonker-Bakker 1991; Sakheim and Devine 1992; Shaffer and Cozolino 1992; Sinanon 1994; Snow and Sorensen 1990; Tate 1991; Van Benschoten 1990; Young et al. 1991). Unfortunately, a strong division exists between believers and nonbelievers. In the Netherlands, disbelief has been reinforced by self-proclaimed experts such as Rossen (1991, 1992), who reduced the Oude Pekela affair to an incident of mass hysteria, and, more recently, by proponents of false memory syndrome.

Aversive reactions of nonbelievers have not affected some therapists in the Netherlands who believe that their patients are genuine child or adult SCSs. However, these therapists are not treating patients in an environment in which SRA is recognized and accepted as a criminal and serious phenomenon that needs to be addressed. Clinicians and the general public do recognize incest as an evil phenomenon, but attacks by the mass media on the validity of incest complaints, as well as a number of controversial incest cases in Dutch courts, have negatively affected the chance that severely abused children will receive proper treatment for SRA and protection from their abusers. In this context, adequate care for child SCSs has become increasingly difficult.

The division between clinicians who take signs and symptoms of SRA seriously and skeptics cannot yet be reconciled because it is difficult to obtain corroborating evidence of SRA (Lanning 1991; J. M. Mulhern 1991; S. Mulhern 1991; Putnam 1991). As Hammond (1992) pointed out, critics tend to overlook the physical evidence that has been found in a number of cases. Some critics allege that clinicians believe SRA exists only because they are being converted to a specific belief system (J. M. Mulhern 1991; Putnam 1991). According to this view, a few zealots are indoctrinating susceptible fellow clinicians in workshops and training seminars on SRA. Dutch clinicians finding SRA cases similar to those reported by North American colleagues therefore must be seen as credulous victims of this indoctrination.

It is true that Dutch clinicians obviously have learned much about SRA from American colleagues. Dutch clinicians believe they finally have been helped to understand artwork (e.g., drawings), signs, symptoms (e.g., observed episodes of reactivated traumatic memories), and behaviors of patients that were present long before they had ever heard of SRA. In most cases, accounts of SRA have been given independently and spontaneously by adults and children from all over the Netherlands.

Conversely, as mentioned before, Dutch clinicians occasionally have met patients who seemed too eager to report SRA. These patients did not show restraint in reporting SRA as did other SCSs, did not seem to be coerced not to discuss SRA, and did not experience the intense anxiety and time-related triggering phenomena or the somatic and other symptoms that more typically seem to be associated with those who appear to be SCSs. In addition, treatment did not proceed as it commonly does in SRA cases. Personality disorders, such as histrionic or narcissistic personality disorder, seemed to be more dominant than severe dissociative symptomatology in patients eager to report SRA. In such cases, credibility is clearly an issue between patient and therapist.

However, hiding our heads in the sand like ostriches will not make SRA go away; it is "better to investigate ritual abuse than to ignore or deny it" (Shaffer 1992). For the sake of SRA patients and their burdened therapists, every attempt should be made to bridge the chasm between them and the skeptics or nonbelievers of SRA.

Those who disbelieve the validity of SRA tend to downplay the scarce legal evidence that does exist. Thus, Tate (1994) reports several British cases in which individuals have been convicted for sadistic sexual abuse within a satanic context. And in Greece, two men received in life sentences for satanic ritual murders (Van Hasselt 1995). According to the charges, the group of satanists to which these two men belonged carried out rituals in tribute to a satanic god—rituals mostly involving drinking and orgies. The *International Herald Tribune* reported the group restrained their victims with chains and handcuffs, tortured them, and in two cases killed them with daggers and a gun (Anastasi 1993). As possibly exemplified in the Dutch Den Helder case mentioned earlier in this chapter, in cases of organized sadistic sexual abuse, often the satanic aspects are downplayed or ignored.

The case of Renee O., a 39-year-old Swiss man arrested in Amsterdam in 1993, is also of interest. On six videotapes that the police found in his Amsterdam residence, the perpetrator was shown sadistically abusing three children, ages 6 months, 18 months, and 12 years. Also found was a wide variety of medical instruments ordinarily used by gynecologists and pediatricians. In his car trunk handcuffs were found. His apartment, in a former satanist church in Amsterdam, contained an aquarium with piranhas, and his house in Switzerland had a tank filled with hydrochloric acid that also contained some remnants of bones.

Although some evidence of his being connected with an international ring of perpetrators existed, Renee O. was regarded by the authorities, including a forensic expert, as an ordinary psychopath acting on his own. We believe that this perpetrator also should have been screened for a dissociative disorder and for possible links with groups involved in SRA.

In heated debates regarding traumatic memories in general and SRA in particular, Dutch trauma therapists, like their North American colleagues, have become targets of vicious attacks. In this hostile climate, it has become even more difficult to treat patients reporting SRA. A forum supported by mental health organizations to discuss problems with respect to patients reporting SRA would be extremely helpful for therapists burdened by the treatment of these extremely traumatized patients. Although we accept that there are various situations that can lead to false and misinterpreted reports of ritual abuse, we have presented accounts from Europe that we believe compel the medical and legal profession to pay attention to the very real possibility that some reports of ritual abuse may be true. The false memory debates have allowed us to become more critical in our assessment and understanding of patients claiming SRA. But our becoming more critical in assessing SRA patients must not deter us from helping real victims of pedophilic and pornographic crimes perpetrated in contrived satanic ceremonies.

References

Aldridge-Morris R: Multiple Personality: An Exercise in Deception. Hillsdale, NJ, Lawrence Erlbaum, 1989

American Psychiatric Association: Diagnostic and Statistical Manual of Mental Disorders, 4th Edition. Washington, DC, American Psychiatric Association, 1994

Anastasi P: Greek satanist group accused of killing 2. International Herald Tribune, December 30, 1993

Bartlett N: Facing the unbelievable. Community Care, December 1989, pp 14–16

Boon S, Draijer N: Diagnosing dissociative disorders in the Netherlands: a pilot study with the Structured Clinical Interview for DSM-III-R dissociative disorders. Am J Psychiatry 148:458–462, 1991

Boon S, Draijer N: Multiple personality disorder in the Netherlands: a clinical investigation of 71 patients. Am J Psychiatry 150:489–494, 1993a

Boon S, Draijer N: Multiple Personality Disorder in the Netherlands: A Study on Reliability and Validity of the Diagnosis. Amsterdam/ Lisse, Swets en Zeitlinger, 1993b

Boon S, van der Hart O: De behandeling van de multiple persoonlijkheids stoornis (Treatment of multiple personality disorder), in Trauma, Dissociatie en Hypnose. Edited by van der Hart O. Lisse, Swets en Zeitlinger, 1995, pp 187–232

Cohen P: Notts team allege sex abuse cover-up. Social Work Today, February 15, 1990, p 3

Crombach H, Merckelbach H: Verdrongen Herinneringen en Andere Misverstanden (Recovered Memories and Other Misunderstandings). Amsterdam, Contact, 1996

Dawson J, Johnston C: When the truth hurts. Community Care, March 30, 1989, pp 11–13

Ellenberger HF: The Discovery of the Unconscious. New York, Basic Books, 1970

Fahy T: Multiple personality disorder (letter). Br J Psychiatry 156:906, 1990

Finkelhor D, Williams L, Burns N: Sexual Abuse in Day Care: A National Study. Durham, NH, Family Research Laboratory, 1988

Fröhling U: Vater Under in der Hölle. Ein Tatsachenbericht Seelze-Velber, Kallmeyer'sche Verlagsbuchhandlung, 1996

Ganaway G: Historical truth versus narrative truth: clarifying the role of exogenous trauma in the etiology of multiple personality disorder and its variants. Dissociation 2:205–220, 1989

Gould C: Satanic ritual abuse: child victims, adult survivors, system response. California Psychologist 22:76–92, 1987

Gould C, Cozolino L: Ritual abuse, multiplicity and mind-control. Journal of Psychology and Theology 20:194–196, 1992

Greaves G: Alternative hypothesis regarding claims of satanic cult activity: a critical analysis, in Out of Darkness: Exploring Satanism and Ritual Abuse. Edited by Sakheim DK, Devine SE. New York, Lexington Books, 1992, pp 45–72

Groenendijk I, van der Hart O: Treatment of DID and DDNOS patients in a regional institute for ambulatory mental health care in the Netherlands: a survey. Dissociation 8:73–83, 1995

Hammond DC: Clinical hypnosis in the treatment of multiple personality disorder. Workshop presented at the Fourth Annual Eastern Regional Conference on Abuse and Multiple Personality Disorder, Alexandria, VA, June 25–29, 1992

Hill S, Goodwin J: Satanism: similarities between patient accounts and pre-Inquisition historical sources. Dissociation 2:39–44, 1989

Hollingsworth J: Unspeakable Acts. New York, Congdon & Weed, 1986

Horevitz R, Loewenstein RJ: The rational treatment of multiple personality disorder, in Dissociation: Clinical and Theoretical Perspectives. Edited by Lynn SJ, Rhue JW. New York, Guilford, 1994, pp 289–316

Huber M: Multiple Persönlichkeiten: Überlebenden Extremer Gewalt (Multiple Personalities: Survivors of Extreme Violence). Frankfurt, Fischer Taschenbuch Verlag, 1995

Hudson P: Ritual Child Abuse, 2nd Edition. Saratoga, CA, R & E Publishers, 1991

Jonker F, Jonker-Bakker P: Experiences with ritualistic child sexual abuse: a case study from the Netherlands. Child Abuse Negl 15:191–196, 1991

Jonker F, Jonker-Bakker P: Reaction to Benjamin Rossen's investigation of satanic ritual abuse in Oude Pekela. Journal of Psychology and Theology 20:260–263, 1992a

Jonker F, Jonker-Bakker P: Safe behind the screen of "mass hysteria": a closing rejoinder to Benjamin Rossen. Journal of Psychology and Theology 20:267–270, 1992b

Kahaner L: Cults That Kill: Probing the Underworld of Occultic Crime. New York, Warner Books, 1988

Karle H: The Filthy Lie. London, Hamish Hamilton, 1992

Kluft RP: Treatment trajectories in multiple personality disorder. Dissociation 7:63–76, 1994

Lanning KV: Ritual abuse: a law enforcement view or perspective. Child Abuse Negl 15:171–173, 1991

Lanning KV: A law enforcement perspective on allegations of ritual abuse, in Out of Darkness: Exploring Satanism and Ritual Abuse. Edited by Sakheim DK, Devine SE. New York, Lexington Books, 1992, pp 109–146

Los Angeles County Commission for Women Ritual Abuse Task Force: Ritual Abuse: Definitions, Glossary, The Use of Mind Control. Los Angeles, CA, Los Angeles County Commission for Women, September 15, 1989

Macilwain IF: Multiple personality disorder (letter). Br J Psychiatry 161:863, 1992

Mulhern JM: Letter. Child Abuse Negl 15:609–610, 1991

Mulhern S: Satanism and psychotherapy: a rumor in search of an inquisition, in The Satanism Scare. Edited by Richardson JT, Best J, Bromley DG. New York, Aldine de Gruyter, 1991, pp 145–172

Putnam FW: The satanic ritual abuse controversy. Child Abuse Negl 15:175–179, 1991

Pyck K: Mass Hysteria in Oude Pekela. Nederlands Tijdschrift voor Criminologie, 1995

Richardson JT, Best J, Bromley DG (eds): The Satanism Scare. New York, Aldine de Gruyter, 1991

Rossen B: Mass hysteria in Oude Pekela. Issues in Child Abuse Accusations 1:49–51, 1991

Rossen B: Response to the Oude Pekela incident and the accusations of Drs. F. Jonker and P. Jonker-Bakker. Journal of Psychology and Theology 20:263–266, 1992

Sakheim DK, Devine SE (eds): Out of Darkness: Exploring Satanism and Ritual Abuse. New York, Lexington Books, 1992

Shaffer RE: Better to investigate ritual abuse than to ignore or deny it: Shaffer responds to Ganaway. Journal of Psychology and Theology 20:208–209, 1992

Shaffer RE, Cozolino LJ: Adults who report childhood ritualistic abuse. Journal of Psychology and Theology 20:188–193, 1992

Sinanon V (ed): Treating Survivors of Satanist Abuse. London, Routledge, 1994

Snow B, Sorensen T: Ritualistic child abuse in a neighborhood. Journal of Interpersonal Violence 5:474–487, 1990

Tate T: Children for the Devil: Ritual Abuse and Satanic Crime. London, Methuen, 1991

Tate T: Press, politics and paedophilia: a practitioner's guide to the media, in Treating Survivors of Satanist Abuse. Edited by Sinanon V. London, Routledge, 1994, pp 182–194

Van Benschoten SC: Multiple personality disorder and satanic ritual abuse: the issue of credibility. Dissociation 3:22–30, 1990 van der Hart O: Multiple personality disorder in Europe: impressions. Dissociation 6:102–118, 1993

van der Hart O, Boon S: Contemporary interest in multiple personality disorder and child abuse in the Netherlands. Dissociation 3:34–37, 1990

van der Hart O, Boon S: Multiple persoonlijkheidsstoornis bij kinderen (Multiple personality disorder in children), in Psychotrauma's bij jongeren (Psychotraumas in youngsters). Edited by Wolters WHG. Baarn, The Netherlands, Ambo, 1991, pp 47–70

Van Hasselt E: Griekse kerk buit "duivelse" moorden uit (Greek Church exploits devilish murders). NRC/Handelsblad, August 8, 1995, p 4

Young WC: Recognition and treatment of survivors reporting ritual abuse, in Out of Darkness: Exploring Satanism and Ritual Abuse. Edited by Sakheim DK, Devine SE. New York, Lexington Books, pp 249–278

Young WC, Sachs RG, Braun BG, et al: Patients reporting ritual abuse in childhood: a clinical syndrome: report of 37 cases. Child Abuse Negl 15:181–189, 1991

Section II

Special Techniques and Issues

Pharmacological Guidelines for Sadistically Abused Patients: From Routine to Critical Issues

Bennett G. Braun, M.D.

*B*efore beginning a discussion of medications for sadistically abused patients, I would like to share a cautionary tale. A young woman was referred to me for evaluation. Her treating clinician described in detail her story related to abuse by a satanic cult and her current eating disorder, anorexia, which he felt was being exacerbated by unresolved issues related to alleged cannibalism. Before her referral to me, her clinician had been treating the anorexia with abreaction after abreaction, trying to work through her memories of cannibalism. The young woman I admitted to the dissociative disorders unit was starving to death. She had to be transferred to a medical floor where she received a central line (subclavian catheter) for parenteral hyperalimentation (forced feeding), which stabilized her physiological and mental condition. After she was stable, evaluation quickly showed that this was a patient with major depression; the driving force behind the anorexia was the depression, not the cannibalism. I found myself treating the patient first for the life-threatening medical condition (starvation), then for the major depression. When asked later if she was a ritual abuse patient, I had to stop and think before replying, so focused was I on keeping this young woman alive and controlling the psychological disorder, depression, that was exacerbating all other symptomatology and preventing any meaningful psychotherapy.

This case is but one of many I have seen where the focus of therapy has been on the horrifying stories exclusively and not on the patient's medical and other psychological problems. For this reason, an explanation of basic medical and psychological evaluation needs to supersede a discussion of medications for sadistically abused patients. The term *sadistic* rather than *ritual abuse* has been chosen. Although ritual abuse has become the catchall descriptor for severe, methodical abuse techniques, it lacks the medical and psychological foundation so essential to formulating a good diagnosis and treatment program. Goodwin's (1993) proposal that clinicians think in terms of sadism and sadistic abuse is a valid one. If patients report they have been beaten, hung from hooks by their wrists, forced to drink abrasive chemicals, and penetrated with foreign objects, then evaluation for physical injury as well as psychological trauma is necessary.

All too often a discussion of psychopharmacological regimens for sadistically abused patients quickly becomes a discussion of medications for dissociative disorder patients, especially those diagnosed with dissociative disorder not otherwise specified (DDNOS) and multiple personality disorder (MPD). This approach is limiting for several reasons, among them the fact that all severely abused patients do not have DDNOS or MPD, and because the approach encourages clinicians to focus on the control of dissociative episodes when they should be continually evaluating their patients' medical and psychological problems.

When treating a sadistically abused patient, the clinician is faced with a problem of separateness in the literature. Over the years, clinicians working with survivors of severe man-made massive trauma, be it Nazi persecution, political torture, or family violence, have developed their own literature to describe the etiology, diagnosis, and treatment of that particular type of trauma. Compounding the problem is the resurgence of the diagnosis dissociative disorder, especially MPD, now called dissociative identity disorder (DID; American Psychiatric Association 1994). Today's clinician treating an alleged ritual abuse patient may find torture, multiplicity, and family violence all in the same patient's diagnostic picture. Although some characteristics of each grouping of trauma must remain unique to that particular group, overall lessons and approaches can benefit the clinician treating ritual abuse patients. In many cases, responding to the triad of symptoms of posttraumatic stress disorder (PTSD)—intrusion, avoidance, and arousal (American Psychiatric Association 1994), with dissociative episodes being one facet of this symptomatology—is the most useful approach to take.

However, life-threatening medical disorders and significant medical problems should be addressed before tackling PTSD's triad. Attention then should focus on immediate, severe behavioral problems. When these problems are under control, then and only then should major psychotherapy be started. If a patient's behavior is out of control, then insight-oriented psychotherapy will only exacerbate the behavior and escalate fear and acting out. Clinicians must corral the behavior (e.g., suicide, acting out, and, in the case of MPD, splitting). In essence, if a patient's physiology is not in proper balance, then all the psychotherapy in the world will not work. For example, an anorexic patient who is starving is unable to concentrate or encode information properly and therefore unable to learn or change behavior.

Any pharmacological regimen also should address the physical, then the psychological. Medications should be used only as adjunctive therapy to control, alleviate, or remove medical and psychological barriers to proper psychotherapy, not as a magic bullet to cure (Braun 1991).

Initial Evaluation

Evaluation of the sadistically abused patient should be approached in the following sequence: 1) physiological, 2) neurophysiological, and 3) psychiatric (behavioral and then psychodynamic) (Braun 1991).

A comprehensive medical examination by an internist skilled in evaluating and treating trauma victims is one of the first steps to building a diagnostic profile from which a medical and psychological treatment plan can be developed. It has been my experience that patients who have been abused since infancy or early childhood do not have a history of consistent medical treatment. Many have not had a complete medical examination in years. Therefore, the initial medical examination can provide both medical and psychological information never before documented.

Clinicians need to be sensitive to the fact that these severely abused patients also can have problems and disorders that do not have a traumatic etiology. Possibilities that should be considered include preexisting genetic disorders; childhood diseases such as rheumatic fever; and predispositions to, or congenital disorders of, cancer, neurodegenerative diseases such as multiple sclerosis, and psychological disorders such as depression and schizophrenia.

Many patients report invasive or confining tortures. It is in the patient's best interest that all medical procedures, especially those requiring invasive techniques, not be performed before the patient has been adequately psychologically prepared for the procedure.

Physiological

A comprehensive medical examination should include the following components:

- An accurate history of the patient's past and present medical condition and medications
- A complete physical examination
- Appropriate laboratory work (including blood, electrocardiogram [ECG], urinalysis, and other tests as indicated)

Many traumatized patients have physical injuries and medical problems. These injuries may have healed improperly or may have left the patient with early-onset, long-term problems, as is seen in early-onset arthritis and bursitis in old joint injuries. In too many cases, legitimate medical problems are dismissed as body memories or somatic memories. Clinicians need to be careful not to label the patient's problems as somatic memories too early in therapy.

It is common for sadistically abused patients to have multisystem disorders stemming from the original trauma, previously undiagnosed genetic predispositions, or lack of medical care. These patients also can have a single disorder with both physical and psychological etiologies. For example, a patient with a history of abuse is being treated for a herniated disc with proper physical therapy and medication for low-back pain and muscle spasms. The patient's problem is not responding completely to these therapies. Then and only then should the clinician think about the perpetuating factor for the complications as being the memory of a traumatic event. If this assumption proves to be accurate, then treatment must be provided at the physical and psychological level simultaneously. The patient may require medications to treat low-back pain on a physical level (muscle relaxants to alleviate muscle spasms; anti-inflammatories and analgesics to relieve pain) and on a psychological level (tranquilizers to relieve anxiety; antidepressants to reduce both pain and depression). Clinicians should be alert to potential drug interactions both between medications and with the psychodynamics of the patient.

Coordination of care by a single physician, often a psychiatrist or internist, is essential when the patient is being cared for by many specialists throughout the course of treatment. However, all clinicians involved in the care of a patient with multisystem disorders should be aware of the medical and psychological problems exhibited by the patient and the possibility of drug interactions causing some of these problems. One of the most effective, efficient ways to coordinate the complex care of these traumatized patients on an outpatient basis is to create outpatient staffings that are similar to staffings on an inpatient unit. This coordination of care is best accomplished with conference calls. The calls not only give clinicians the opportunity to share progress reports and plan future treatment directions, but also have the added benefit of providing teaching opportunities among the specialties (Braun 1991).

Neurophysiological

Because amnesia to traumatic events can be one of the main features of any trauma, a differential diagnosis of memory problems is essential (Putnam 1989). For example, are we seeing a true dementia, a pseudodementia, repression of information, or blocking due to severe anxiety?

If the patient is experiencing a true seizure disorder, then the differential diagnosis for pseudoseizure must be made, allowing for the possibility of both being present. Because electroencephalogram (EEG) focuses only on a time when seizure activity may not be present, one may, if possible, draw a blood sample for a prolactin level immediately after the seizure and then again a half hour later. A true seizure generally shows a doubling or more in prolactin level.

Many patients who have experienced severe trauma or abuse complain of headaches. Headaches can have physiological and/or psychological etiologies. Physiological etiologies include tumor, vascular insufficiency, increased intracranial pressure, and severe head injury. Depression, internalized aggression, anxiety, and unexpressed anger can lead to headaches with psychological underpinnings. A differential diagnosis must be made, recognizing both the physiological and psychological manifestations of headache (Braun 1983; Braun et al. 1992). A brain tumor or neurodegenerative diseases also can account for loss of memory, decreased muscle tone, and specific or nonspecific pain. Migraine headaches too can have a physiological and/or psychological basis and precipitants.

General Comments on Medications

In the remainder of this chapter, I discuss general guidelines for using psychopharmacological agents in treating severely traumatized patients, as well as specific interventions for commonly found symptoms. I discuss basic principles so that the prescribing physician will have a starting point, the nonphysician will be able to appreciate what is being done, and they both will be able to ask intelligent questions about indications and contraindications of commonly used medications. They can then question whether the current symptom is trauma based or medication based.

Several useful resources are available to clinicians who want an understanding of basic pharmacology and clinical drug use: *The Pharmacologic Basis of Therapeutics* (Goodman and Gilman 1985), *Manual of Clinical Psychopharmacology*, Third Edition (Schatzberg et al. 1997), and *Pharmacology in Nursing* (Hahn et al. 1986). *Physicians' Desk Reference* (PDR), published annually by Medical Economics Data, describes individual medications and their indications and contraindications.

In general, medications can be useful in managing PTSD symptoms in the following ways:

- To decrease the general hyperarousal and vigilance that characterize the syndrome
- To promote improved sleep and to control nightmares
- To provide greater distance between the patient and the emotional impact of the trauma
- To improve the patient's mood and relieve depression, suicidality, and anhedonia
- To enhance control over impulses of aggression and violence
- To control psychotic manifestations when these are present (Davidson 1991)

Medication is not the definitive treatment for these patients; psychotherapy generally is. Medication is titrated according to the symptoms so that the psychotherapy can be done.

General guidelines for administering medications are as follows:

- No patient should be given medications before a complete history and medical examination has been performed.
- Medications for potentially life-threatening medical problems and behaviors take priority over medications to relieve psychological distress.
- Psychopharmacology for psychological distress should be considered only to alleviate symptoms and only with the knowledge that many patients will not require psychopharmacological medications after they have completed appropriate psychotherapy, or medication may need to be reduced or stopped after significant issues have been worked through.
- Patients with multisystem problems usually require a variety of medications to control symptoms. Therefore, there may be potential adverse drug interactions. For example, when patients take clonazepam (Klonopin, Rivotril), carbamazepine (Tegretol), and tricyclic antidepressants at the same time, they suddenly may become ataxic due to the combined effect on the cerebellum.
- Severely traumatized patients often use avoidance and dissocia-

tion as major psychological defenses. Patients taking anxiolytics, sedatives, hypnotics, and analgesics should be monitored closely because they may ask for increased doses of these medications to achieve a chemical dissociation.

- Many psychopharmacological agents and analgesic medications have addictive properties that can lead to abuse and addiction in patients who, in many cases, are already troubled by substance abuse problems (Putnam 1989).

- Some patients report being drugged as part of their childhood abuse. Loewenstein (1991) describes various reactions to psychotropic medications:

> [Patients] may react post-traumatically to various aspects of being prescribed medications. This can include recalling or reliving childhood drug reactions to agents said to be similar to those currently being prescribed. Conversion and spontaneous flashbacks may occur in this context. Sometimes this can lead to confusion in evaluating an apparent drug reaction. Occasionally the patient will become so "triggered" by aspects of taking psychotropic medications that any beneficial effect of the drug is confounded. (p. 726)

- Generally, medications should be administered using the guidelines approved by the U.S. Food and Drug Administration (FDA). Use of pharmacological agents outside of the guidelines must be done with close control and appropriate study and rationale. If a pharmacological agent is to be used outside of the specified guidelines, informed consent must be obtained from the patient. Unusual uses of medications should be accompanied by proper medical monitoring. For example, I have found when propranolol and clonidine are given in much higher than normal doses, they can both decrease anxiety and the frequency of switching of alters (Braun 1991).

Specific Indications and Medications

The following discussions are brief overviews of symptoms commonly seen in severely traumatized patients and useful treatment or medication regimens.

Medical Problems

Severe medical problems must be addressed before any other medical or psychological issues. Acute medical problems, such as congestive heart failure, pulmonary embolism, severe asthma, pneumonia, cardiovascular accident, and appendicitis, need to be treated by appropriate medical standards. It has been stated that in the case of dissociative disorder patients, alter personalities or fragments may respond differently to the same dose of a given medication (Barkin et al. 1986). This finding does not hold for antibiotics, anti-inflammatories, some cardiac medications (digitalis), and others.

Pain. When assessing a complaint of pain, clinicians need to be aware that they may be dealing with a somatic memory or a present-day injury or chronic physical condition. It is also possible that a bout of pain can be precipitated by a real injury but maintained by a somatic memory. Pain is the most common complaint used to obtain medication to achieve chemical dissociation.

First-line analgesics such as aspirin, acetaminophen, and ibuprofen (Motrin) can be used relatively freely if patients are monitored for side effects such as anticoagulation and gastrointestinal tract bleeding and irritation. Second-line analgesics such as codeine and its derivatives need to be used with more caution because of their addicting and constipating effects and ability to cause chemical dissociation. Propoxyphene napsylate (Darvocet-N 100) or naproxen (Naprosyn) may be safer but may not be as effective. Tertiary analgesics such as narcotics or their equivalents must be prescribed with extreme caution because they also are addictive and can cause chemical dissociation. In addition, this third group of medications can precipitate euphoria and decreased concentration and reasoning, all which interfere significantly with any psychotherapeutic progress.

Eating disorders. Eating disorders are considered a medical problem because of their potential serious physiological manifestations, which must take priority over psychological treatment. Only after patients' electrolytic balance and nutritional status have been corrected sufficiently should psychotherapy be considered. When the level of amino acids is insufficient, proper encoding of information cannot take place, rendering psychotherapy useless.

Patients with extreme debilitation may require a subclavian catheter and hyperalimentation. Hyperalimentation can be started on a medical unit and continued on a psychiatric unit if the nurses are properly trained. Tube feedings may be necessary until patients are willing to take nourishment voluntarily. Patients who have trouble eating certain foods because they are reminders of past traumatic episodes may agree to take liquid food supplements and multiple vitamins with minerals. Inpatients who have bulimia need to be kept out of their rooms and monitored for 1.5–2 hours after eating.

When appropriate, naltrexone hydrochloride (Trexan) will facilitate an impressive reduction in bulimic behavior. Other medications that help control obsessive-compulsive behaviors of both bulimia and anorexia are the serotonin and selective serotonin reuptake inhibitors (SRIs and SSRIs) such as clomipramine hydrochloride (Anafranil) and fluoxetine hydrochloride (Prozac).

Seizure disorders. Medications used to control seizure disorders also can be used to treat psychological problems if clinicians choose wisely. Clonazepam may be chosen, if appropriate, over carbamazepine and primidone (Mysoline) because clonazepam not only decreases seizure activity, but also can be used to lie in a base of a long-acting benzodiazepine to help reduce anxiety. On top of this base can be added a short-acting benzodiazepine such as alprazolam (Xanax) or lorazepam (Ativan), both of which have antiseizure qualities.

Substance abuse. Patients who are abusing alcohol or recreational drugs will not respond appropriately to either psychotherapy or medications taken to alleviate other symptomatology such as depression and anxiety. Disulfiram (Antabuse) can be an effective deterrent to drinking, if the patient does not sabotage the effects of the drug through contact with alcohol. Using clonidine (Catapres), benzodiazepines, and other medications to facilitate withdrawal is beyond the scope of this chapter.

Depression

The treatment of depression is often the turning point in the treatment of a sadistically abused patient. If patients are depressed, they have difficulty thinking and making decisions. Difficulty in thinking and decision making, in addition to negativity, often renders psychotherapy ineffective. In the treatment schema, therefore, depression has priority over issues of sadistic abuse or dissociation. If memories of the sadistic abuse are treated before depression is controlled, patients will act out because they are overloaded by internal and external stimuli with which they are unable to cope.

Tricyclic or polycyclic antidepressants are most commonly used to treat depression. Clinicians need to be aware of the side effects of antidepressants, especially when used in combination with other medications. For example, nortriptyline (Pamelor) may further lower blood pressure of a patient receiving a β-blocker such as propranolol (Inderal).

SSRIs are becoming the first-line choice for treating depression because of their effectiveness and more tolerable side-effect profile. Theoretically, SSRIs as a group have the additional benefit, in high doses, of being useful for obsessive-compulsive symptomatology.

Monoamine oxidase inhibitors (MAOIs) are valuable in treating not only resistant depressions, but also panic disorder with or without agoraphobia, and atypical depression, which are seen frequently in sadistically abused patients. Unfortunately, I often have not been able to use MAOIs when I would have liked to because I could not trust the patient to remain on a tyramine-free diet. Some other countries have moclobemide (Manerix) available, a new-generation MAOI (selective, type A), which does not require dietary restrictions as does the original MAOI group. I believed the risk to a patient's health and life was greater from his or her sabotaging the effects of the medication than from depression when the patient was treated with older-generation MAOIs. In those cases, I used an SSRI instead.

Anxiety

Anxiety, another common symptom found in severely traumatized patients, is often treated with benzodiazepines. As a group, benzodiazepines are central nervous system depressants and have sedative and hypnotic properties.

Benzodiazepines are useful in 1) relieving persistent anxiety, 2) facilitating management of recognizable stress, and 3) diminishing recurrent distressing dreams, motor tension, autonomic hyperactivity, apprehensive expectation, vigilance and scanning, persistent and irrational fears, and excessive and unreasonable panic (Allodi 1991; Barkin et al. 1986).

Benzodiazepines have chemical properties that can cause physical and/or psychological addiction. Patients who have been taking high doses of benzodiazepines for long periods may have withdrawal problems if they abruptly stop taking the medication. Chemical dissociation is another frequent complication.

Short- and long-acting benzodiazepines such as alprazolam and clonazepam are commonly prescribed. I have been known to prescribe cautiously four different benzodiazepines for the same patient, using the following rationale: When using a short-acting benzodiazepine, such as alprazolam or lorazepam, a clinician may see a yo-yo effect, wherein the patient's metabolism for the medication accelerates and he or she goes into withdrawal just before the next dose. This yo-yo effect often causes the physician continually to increase the amount of medication, thinking that the patient is taking an insufficient dose. Instead of increasing a short-acting benzodiazepine, I add a long-acting benzodiazepine, such as clonazepam or clorazepate dipotassium (Tranxene), as a base on top of which I titrate a smaller amount of a short-acting benzodiazepine.

Alprazolam is my first choice because it has both antianxiety and antidepressant properties and can be used to augment sedation for sleep. However, it is metabolized by the body much faster than the longer-acting benzodiazepines such as clorazepate or clonazepam. Clonazepam can be used as a long-acting tranquilizer and supplemented with alprazolam to avoid the peaks and valleys seen with long-term administration of shorter-acting benzodiazepines.

Insomnia

Patients may have problems both falling asleep and staying asleep. Sleep problems often are resolved with short-acting benzodiazepines, such as triazolam (Halcion), to help the patient fall asleep quickly and an intermediate-acting benzodiazepine, such as temazepam (Restoril), to help the patient remain asleep. This method of treatment relies on pharmacokinetics. As triazolam is being metabolized out of the system, temazepam is increasing in serum concentration. I do not prescribe a long-acting benzodiazepine such as flurazepam (Dalmane) for insomnia patients because its half-life is approximately 5 days, unless I am also using it as a long-acting anxiolytic and want daytime sedation.

Benzodiazepines classified as sedative or hypnotic include triazolam, temazepam, flurazepam, and lorazepam. They are useful in the short-term management of insomnia characterized by difficulty falling or staying asleep and frequent nocturnal or early-morning awakening, or insomnia secondary to anxiety or transient-situated stresses. These benzodiazepines also chemically may cause a loss of memory. For example, patients may take lorazepam 1 hour before bedtime and then decide to finish a project they are working on; the following day, they may not remember working on that project.

Dissociation

Several good sources are available for clinicians who want information about using psychopharmacological agents in treating MPD patients (Barkin et al. 1986; Braun 1990; Loewenstein 1991; Putnam 1989). All report that medication will not cure a dissociative disorder but will control or alleviate symptoms. To date, there have been no double-blind, controlled medication studies on dissociative disorder patients.

I have found that propranolol and clonidine, when given in doses far in excess of FDA guidelines, reduce personality-state switching in patients with MPD for whom no other therapy has worked (Braun 1990). However, when all other treatment options have been exhausted and excessive doses of the medication are necessary, patients are monitored frequently on an inpatient unit and not discharged until they understand the rationale, side effects, and risks. Patients must be able to 1) take their own blood pressure and pulse, both sitting and standing, and keep proper records; 2) understand and remember not to take a dose of medication if their blood pressure or pulse falls outside of designated limits; and 3) call their physician should problems arise. When patients are able to observe these three guidelines, they can be managed on an outpatient basis (Braun 1990).

Self-Mutilating Behaviors

Sadistically abused patients are often severe self-mutilators. A patient who is self-mutilating should be evaluated and appropriately treated on four levels simultaneously (Braun 1991):

1. Endorphin autoaddiction syndrome, the patient's drug-seeking behavior, focuses on what will get the patient his or her drug—the brain's release of endorphins (Braun 1991). My experience has been that this syndrome is successfully controlled with naltrexone. This drug reduces the reinforcing properties of the endorphin release by selectively blocking the μ receptors, preventing the rush or calm that these patients report and causing the patient to experience pain.
2. Obsessive-compulsive disorder (OCD) responds to SRIs such as clomipramine and fluoxetine.
3. Cognitive distortions and inappropriate coping mechanisms are treated with cognitive therapy and behavior modification.
4. The psychology of perpetuators such as guilt, shame, and fear often needs to be explored using psychodynamic psychotherapy.

Conclusion

Many sadistically abused patients have multisystem problems and disorders requiring the care of many specialists. I have found that in too many cases of severely traumatized patients, medical problems are not diagnosed or, if they are, are treated incorrectly. In this chapter, I introduced some of the more common medical and psychological problems of sadistically abused patients and the pharmacological interventions. I hope this chapter also reminds us that the French developed the only effective method to separate mind and body—the guillotine.

References

Allodi FA: Assessment and treatment of torture victims: a critical review. J Nerv Ment Dis 197:4–11, 1991

American Psychiatric Association: Diagnostic and Statistical Manual of Mental Disorders, 4th Edition. Washington, DC, American Psychiatric Association, 1994

Barkin RL, Braun BG, Kluft RP: The dilemma of drug therapy for multiple personality disorder, in Treatment of Multiple Personality Disorder. Edited by Braun BG. Washington, DC, American Psychiatric Press, 1986, pp 107–132

Braun BG: Psychophysiologic phenomena in multiple personality and hypnosis. Am J Clin Hypn 26:124–137, 1983

Braun BG: Unusual medication regimens in the treatment of dissociative disorder patients, I: noradrenergic agents. Dissociation 3:144–150, 1990

Braun BG: The therapeutic frame: from physiologic to psychologic. Paper presented at the Eighth International Conference on Multiple Personality/Dissociative States, Chicago, IL, November 15–17, 1991

Braun BG, Sachs RG, Frischholz EJ: Headaches and early child abuse: sexual aspects of headaches, in Sexual Aspects of Headaches. Edited by Diamond S, Maliszewski M. Madison, CT, International Universities Press, 1992, pp 379–388

Davidson J: Clinical management of post-traumatic stress disorder, in The Clinical Management of Anxiety Disorders. Edited by Coryell W, Winokur G. New York, Oxford University Press, 1991

Goodman LS, Gilman AG: The Pharmacologic Basis of Therapeutics, 7th Edition. New York, Macmillan, 1985

Goodwin J: Rediscovering sadism (editor's introduction), in Rediscovering Childhood Trauma: Historical Casebook and Clinical Applications. Edited by Goodwin J. Washington, DC, American Psychiatric Press, 1993, pp 89–93

Hahn AB, Barkin RL, Oestreich S: Pharmacology in Nursing, 16th Edition. St. Louis, MO, CV Mosby, 1986

Loewenstein RJ: Rational psychopharmacology in the treatment of multiple personality disorder. Psychiatr Clin North Am 14:721–740, 1991

Putnam FW: Diagnosis and Treatment of Multiple Personality Disorder. New York, Guilford, 1989

Schatzberg AF, Cole JO, DeBattista C (eds): Manual of Clinical Psychopharmacology, Third Edition. Washington, DC, American Psychiatric Press, 1997

CHAPTER 9

Visions of Memories:
A Patient's Visual Representation of
Ritual Abuse Ceremonies

George A. Fraser, M.D., F.R.C.P.C.

Sometimes a picture is worth a thousand words. The artwork included in this chapter was done by a patient who has been in therapy with me. She has given permission to have them published in this book. Except for the first three, the patient drew these pictures during therapy to convey what she believes are her memories of ceremonies in a satanic cult. She believes these memories were withheld by alter personalities who were too frightened to tell but felt safe to convey through drawings. Later, I was able to discuss the drawings with the patient and ask her to explain what they represented. These discussions helped the patient understand the belief system of inner personality states who claimed they had been abused in a satanic cult in perverse and sadistic ways.

I do not know, of course, whether or not the drawings represent true memories. If they do, this is probably the closest most of us will ever get to see satanic ritual ceremonies. Because the drawings portray so well what many therapists are being told, I felt that it would be helpful to include this pictorial chapter.

Caution is necessary before proceeding to read this chapter. Many of the scenes are graphic and represent abusive situations. Reader caution is advised: Some readers may be sensitive and could be upset by the drawings and what they might represent. Those who suspect this chapter might upset them should discuss it with someone who could advise and support them. If in therapy, discuss it first with your therapist before deciding to proceed with this chapter.

In the 1980s, before I had encountered any patients reporting ritual abuse (RA) memories, I received a letter from Europe from a patient whom I was treating for multiple personality disorder. She had suddenly left with her mother to visit relatives in the Netherlands. She was writing to explain why she had missed her sessions with me and why she would likely miss a few more. On the back of her letter were three rather unusual drawings. They certainly caught my attention, but they seemed unrelated to anything we had dealt with in therapy.

When she returned from overseas, I asked her if there was a meaning to the drawings. She seemed puzzled, so I showed them to her. She said they were not hers, and she did not know what they meant. After a while, she said that she now recalled that she had trouble finding writing paper when in Europe and had torn some sheets from a drawing tablet that belonged to an alter personality whom I had never heard of before and was not able to contact when I asked to meet with her.

I didn't think much more of the drawings and dropped the subject. It was a year or two later in therapy when further material came out that had themes suggesting she was involved in a satanic cult and possibly ritually abused.

To the best of my memory, this was my first patient who gave information consistent with stories I had heard indicating RA. It was 1987. As it turns out, she was only the first of a number of patients who gave RA histories. Perhaps because she was one of the first to report recollections of RA in central and eastern Canada, her drawings (circa 1985–1986) can be considered less likely to be contaminated by the subsequent flood of RA reports in the media.

Long after I had received the patient's letter from Europe, when I had dealt with more reports of RA, I returned to the drawings on the back of that letter. Only then did I realize those drawings had themes similar to later drawings I saw produced by patients reporting RA. I had not even considered RA when I first received the letter.

I do not believe I had any influence on the drawings shown here.

Figures 9–4 through 9–9 come from a later phase in the patient's therapy, probably 1990. When I discussed the possibility of using the pictures in this book, the patient gave written permission but became distressed when I wanted her to refresh my memory of what they represented. She said she never wanted to see them again. I have respected this request and have not shown the pictures to her again. I am relying on my recollections of what she had said in therapy some years ago.

I present these drawings to represent pictorially the stories being reported to therapists who struggle with the dilemma of RA. Whether or not some reports are based on abuses with satanic themes, culture-bound fantasies, urban legends, or whatever, we in the psychiatric field nonetheless need to work together to offer the best management for those with recollections of RA.

In Figure 9–1, a young cult member, presumably the patient herself, is being warned that her heart will be torn out of her body while she is alive if she ever reveals what happens in the cult. The eyelike sun is a reminder that no one can escape the ever-watchful eye of Satan. The pyramids represent power. The two on the right themselves are filled with pyramids and eyes. The base of the largest pyramid contains an inverted pyramid with the three crosses of Calvary at the apex. The center cross is an inverted crucifix, supposedly representing a mockery of Christ.

In the foreground of Figure 9–2 are scissors and a butcher knife, instruments said to be used within a cult when bodies are dismembered. In the background is an eye-filled pyramid with a central inverted crucifix at the apex. To the left is a pill container with a medical insignia. In it are pills and a skull and crossbones representing the drugging and poisoning done to the patient, who is trapped within. Her vacant face suggests she awaits emergence of whichever alter personality will be activated by the effect of these drugs.

The kites contain clownlike masks reportedly used in ceremonies to conceal the identities of those involved in cult activities, which frequently are described as sexual orgies.

In the lower right of Figure 9–3 is a cult leader. He carries a staff or mace adorned with an official-looking insignia. I believe the

Figure 9–1

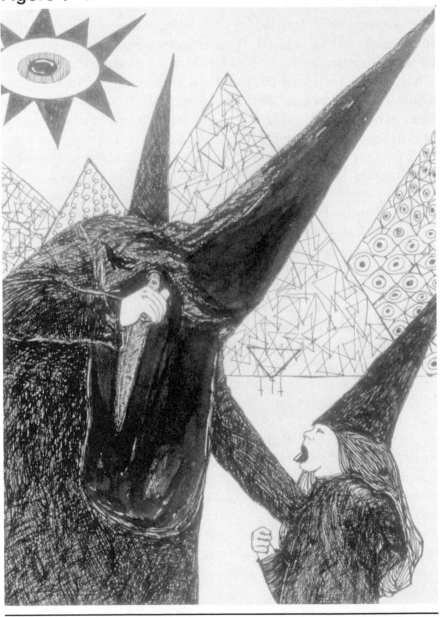

crown on the insignia is similar to that I have seen used to represent royalty. To the bottom left, Calvary is again depicted, along with the inverted cross. I have erased other satanic symbols to avoid possibly identifying the patient and any group to which she may have belonged.

In the middle, to the left, is a torso in the process of being eviscerated. Serpents bite both thighs. This drawing implies that a human sacrifice victim is being disposed of so evidence of this murder will not be found. The torso has "666," the "sign of the beast" (Satan), carved in the left thigh. This drawing might make one wonder if the victim was a cult member.

Dismembered body parts can be seen in the left pyramid, while eyes with perhaps the superimposed sign for anarchy are present in the right pyramid. The central pyramid contains wavy lines, which I recall the patient saying had satanic symbolism. I am uncertain if the white hood has any special meaning as all others are black.

Figure 9–2

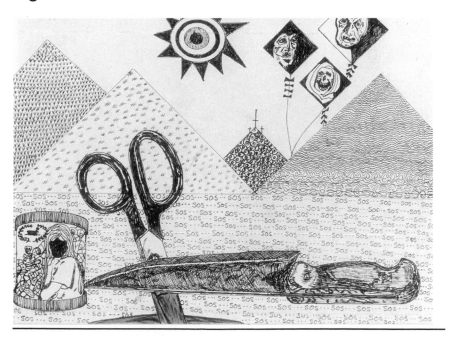

Figure 9–3

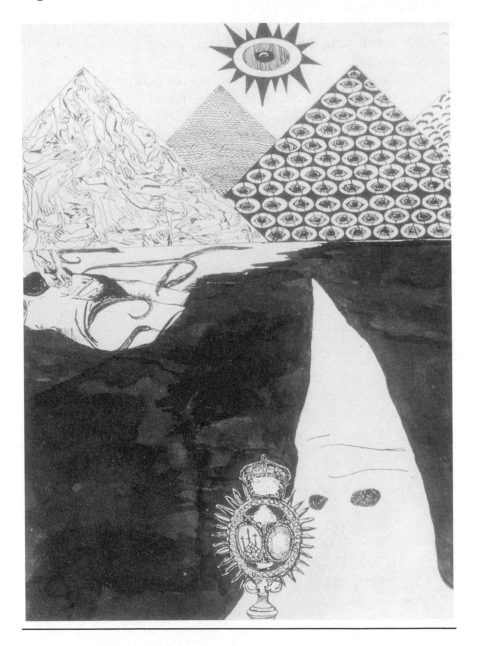

The following drawings (Figures 9–4 through 9–9) were done as part of therapy after the possibility of RA was recognized by the patient. The drawings were not done by the host personality. As we looked at them in therapy, the meaning was told to her by the personality who did the drawings, and she relayed to me what she was being told.

Figure 9–4 depicts someone in prolonged isolation. The patient reported that she was frequently kept in isolation without any of her basic needs being met, including food, drink, and toilet facilities. This isolation could go on for a couple of days. She believes she was isolated so that cult members could force her to submit to any request they made. She says she learned to respond to any request without hesitation and without question. She reported similar isolation when she was a child but said as a child she sometimes was kept in a cage alone or with other children. Her descriptions were similar to writings on mind-coercion techniques illegally used on political prisoners to extract information and cooperation.

In Figure 9–5, body parts are being exhumed during a clandestine meeting in a graveyard. The patient says this shows her as a young girl being forced by a friend of the family, whom she knows is in the cult, to watch a skull being removed from a grave. Although she believed she vomited as she watched in horror, she was still forced to look. Later, a hand from behind was placed directly on her face as a sign, often repeated, that what she saw was never to be revealed. Whenever she subsequently saw a hand with the palm facing her, it was said to be a signal reminding her never to tell what she had seen and experienced.

The patient says Figure 9–6 depicts a ritual ceremony in which she was impregnated. Her child was to be used for whatever reason desired by the cult. There would be about a half-dozen participants in this impregnation so that the identity of the father would not be known. Patients who report this ritual have said they are called *cult breeders*. The "gentleman" in the center appears ready to be the first participant as he begins by letting blood from her wrist with a ceremonial dagger. The drawing suggests sexual sadism, including bondage and voyeurism.

The bodies floating above the altar were said to be previously formed personality states who are sequentially dissociating to an

Figure 9–4

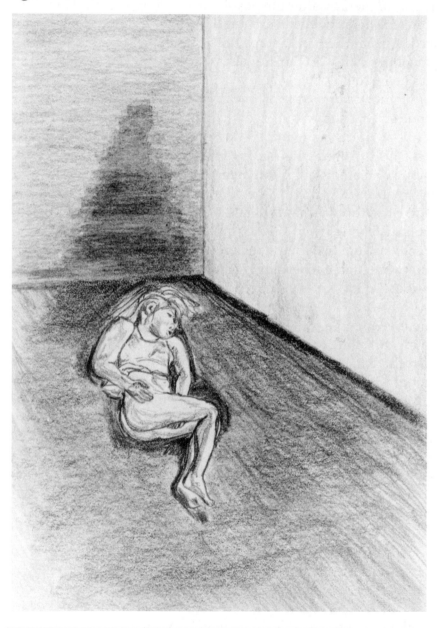

Figure 9–5

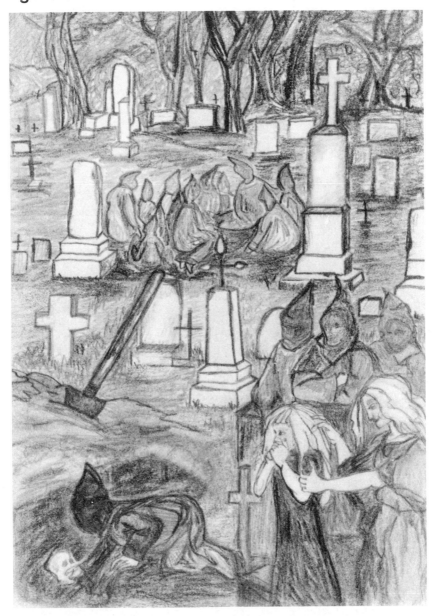

Figure 9–6

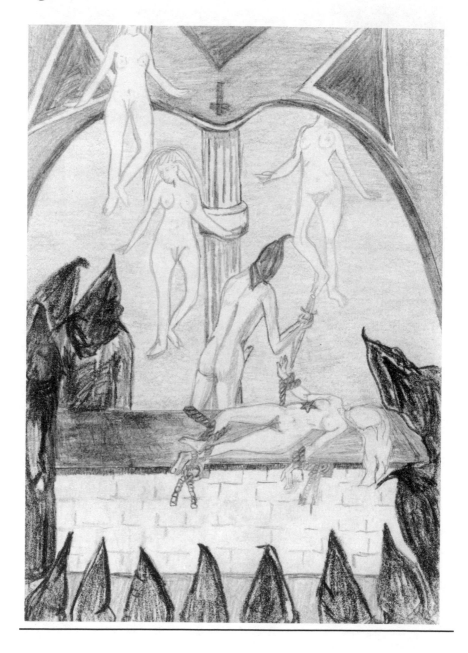

out-of-body experience. In a very real sense, the last personality left is the one who will experience the abuse. This picture shows a blank face, suggesting the initiation of a new personality state: one who was likely to be present for all future "breeding ceremonies." The other personalities would either have amnesia or at the most a remote feeling of having observed the event from a distance, with little emotional connection.

In Figure 9–7, the pregnancy has reached term. The raised sword will not kill the patient but will be used to let blood, which will be placed in a chalice and drunk by the participating hooded members. Drinking of blood is commonly reported. Many satanic rituals or ceremonies are said to be variations on those of Christian services.

She reported that dildos, birds, and snakes are inserted, even at the later stages of pregnancy. Again, the patient's drawing suggests that sexual gratification, sadism, and perversion are central to the ceremonies.

A 666 is noted on the left thigh. The physician who performed the physical examination when the patient was an inpatient confirmed scarring consistent with this pattern of numbers on her inner left thigh.

Figure 9–8 shows a child engaged in an initiation ceremony; this child already has been selected to be an adult member of the cult. A chalice is noted on the left of the altar. The scene has overtones of a religious ceremony.

In a scene somewhat similar to that in Figure 9–8, the patient portrays herself as an older child going through an important ritualistic ceremony in Figure 9–9. She is in the center of a circle formed by burning candles. There has been some bloodletting, and sticks are carefully inserted into every orifice while chants are sung by participants. I recall the patient said that her body was in alignment with certain points of the compass during this ceremony.

The patient said that the high priest, on attaining that rank, would ceremoniously cut off the distal part of his left middle finger. The amputated finger was a very powerful symbol of leadership.

A hypodermic needle is noted to the right. The patient said injections were given to produce an altered or dissociated state in a child. This patient had once bragged to me that she knew how to make a multiple personality in a child. I asked her to explain. She

Figure 9–7

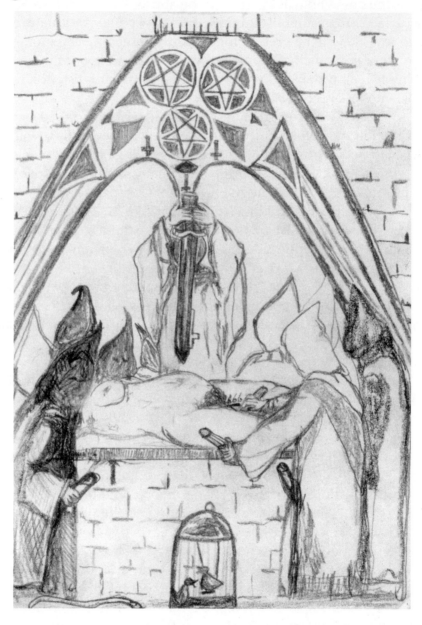

Figure 9–8

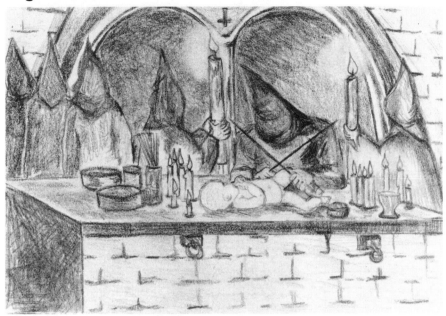

answered that first you take a child and confine it in a box. Then you add worms, bugs, and snakes and place a lid on the box. The child will kick and scream in terror. You ignore the child until no noise comes from the box, at which time you remove the top of the box. You then check the muscle tone of the child. If the tone is relaxed, you have caused a dissociated switch, and you can now train this new personality to be who you want and to do what you want. The child will obey without question. Her explanation was quite unsettling to hear because it just might work if the child has a high capacity for dissociation.

These drawings represent some of the events and abuse reported to therapists by patients who believe they have participated in RA groups. The drawings vividly depict ritualistic ceremonies and ways in which those in therapy claim they have been terrorized. Although the pictures are realistic and graphic, they do not prove they portray actual events. Conversely, one also must consider the possibility that these drawings reveal memories of witnessed and experienced events.

Figure 9–9

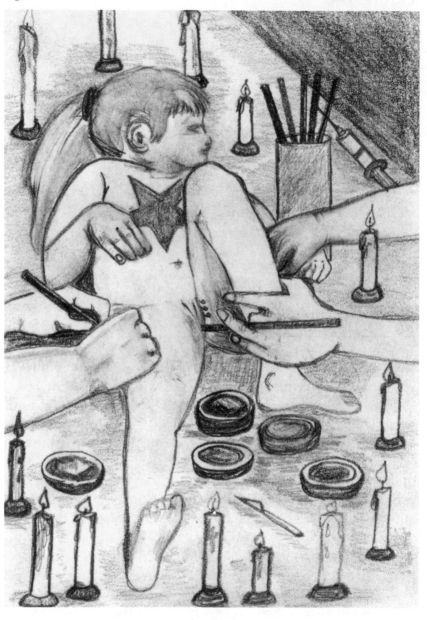

The Court System and the Problem of Hypnotically Recovered Memories: A Forensic Psychiatrist's Concerns

John M. W. Bradford, M.D., F.R.C.P.C.

I have been observing the phenomenon of ritualized sexual abuse and the sometimes related debate over false memories from a different viewpoint than most readers of this book. I am a forensic psychiatrist who is often called as an expert witness in the courtroom, not for victims of sexual abuse but more often in relationship to the perpetrators of these sadistic sexual abuses. From this vantage point, I see errors being made by some therapists appearing on behalf of patients who were allegedly victims of ritual abuse (RA). The courtroom is a very different environment from the therapy room. The rules that govern one are often foreign to the other.

Therapists are often unaware of the rules pertaining to court hearings. They frequently appear as expert witnesses, although they are unqualified to do so. Often, the only reason they are called as expert witnesses is to present uncorroborated evidence they obtained through sometimes leading questioning techniques that uncovered long-lost memories of sexual abuses in their patients. Usually, therapists are totally ignorant of courts' rules on the admissibility of hypnotically enhanced memories, whether they are found through formal or informal hypnotic techniques.

In this chapter, I discuss RA with the hope of informing therapists about some of the potential pitfalls to be considered before rushing RA cases before a judge and jury.

Consider Pitfalls Before Rushing to the Courtroom

Having spent the past 14 years of my life working principally with perpetrators of child sexual abuse, I am sensitive to the controversy surrounding RA. First, there is a complete polarization of groups who support victims versus those who assess and treat perpetrators. Further, there is a group who believe that ritualized sexual abuse of women and children exists and another group who just as firmly believe that RA is completely nonexistent. The significant issue is that RA is a matter of beliefs, and these beliefs are of dubious scientific value.

Another factor influencing the RA controversy is that ritualized sexual exploitation of women and children recently has received enormous media coverage, driven by ritualized sexual abuse in day care starting with the McMartin case in Manhattan Beach, California, and followed by similar cases elsewhere in the United States and Canada. Cases of ritualized sexual abuse capture the attention of the media and subsequently that of the public. In a number of these cases, ritualized sexual abuse has been discredited. The Eileen Franklin case initially appeared to lend enormous credit to delayed memory recall when, 20 years after her father allegedly had murdered her best friend, she looked down at her own daughter's face and started to recall the events of the day of the murder. Specific corroborating evidence appeared to substantiate the accuracy of her delayed memories. This case has now been reported extensively in both the print and visual media and is documented in an excellent book (Franklin and Wright 1993). However, by the mid-1990s, the courts began questioning convictions based solely on uncorroborated recovered memories. In 1995, a California federal judge overturned Franklin's conviction.

Lanning (1992), a supervisory special agent in the U.S. Federal Bureau of Investigation (FBI) Behavioral Science Unit, led investigations of RA and reported that beginning in the early 1980s stories of satanic rituals began emerging. These stories included sexual victimization of women and children in satanic sacrifices. This type of abuse was later referred to as "ritual" sexual abuse.

Case reports of RA grew, with allegations of hundreds, perhaps thousands, of victims being murdered in organized satanic cults. The FBI and other law enforcement agencies extensively investigated these allegations for approximately 8 years and found very little evidence to support satanic ritualized abuse. Specifically, there was no corroboration of baby breeding for human sacrifice and other satanic activities. In fact, other than the discoveries of murders in Matamoros, Mexico, in 1989, which did involve satanic and ritualized murder, there is no other evidence in the FBI's investigations. Lanning (1991, 1992) emphasizes that if one thinks logically about the practical difficulties of hiding the physical evidence of ritualized murders, preventing people from talking (because in large groups there is always some dissenter who would want to expose the satanic activities), and other factors, it is impossible that large-scale ritualized sexual or nonsexual abuse exists.

Like Lanning, I was having difficulty believing these stories. In my experience as a forensic psychiatrist and the director of a highly developed sexual behaviors clinic, I have assessed thousands of sexual offenders, many of whom were pedophiles, and studied lie detection and the phenomenon of dissociative amnesia in forensic psychiatric patients. I have become painfully aware of the ignorance and confusion about these issues among mental health professionals. There appears to be a number of therapists with little professional training and poor credentials whom I suspect understand little about transference, suggestibility, and other important issues related to the therapeutic interaction. These individuals, as a result of their interaction with patients and ignorance as to what damage they are doing, have contaminated the minds of patients consulting them. They have confused fact and fantasy in the minds of their patients and appear to have created pseudomemories and other difficulties generating fantastic claims of satanic rituals.

Paraphilias:
A Multiplicity of Deviant Behaviors

Conversely, I have in at least one study (Bradford et al. 1992) shown
the enormous extent of sexually deviant activity perpetrated
against women and both prepubertal and adolescent children. The
perpetrators have not just one sexual deviation, but multiple
paraphilias. In addition, these paraphilias cross over so that one
perpetrator has a number of techniques to victimize vulnerable
women and children. Colleagues (Abel et al. 1985) also have shown
the vast extent of paraphilic behavior in a study of more than 400
paraphilic men. A study by Timnick (1985) and the *Los Angeles Times*
showed that between 10.9 and 17.6 million American men have
sexually abused a child and that 27% of females and 16% of males
were victims of sexual assaults. Based on a Gallup survey of more
than 2,000 Canadians, the Badgely Committee (Committee on Sexual Offences Against Children and Youths 1984) reported that one
in two females and one in three males were victims of unwanted
sexual acts when they were children or youths. The acts included
a spectrum of sexual abuse behaviors, but of concern was the degree
of coercion and force reported. Sixty percent of these children and
adolescents were threatened or physically coerced during the unwanted sexual acts (Committee on Sexual Offences Against Children and Youths 1984). These accurate and scientifically valid
studies support the contention that ritualized sexual abuse must
occur and that when a problem is so extensive, it can be regarded
as a serious public health problem in the United States and Canada.
Further, many priests have been charged with and pleaded guilty
to sexual abuse with, on occasion, a background of religious rituals,
sadistic beatings, and coercion, incidents supporting the existence
of what could be termed ritualized sexual abuse. An estimated 2%–
6% of Roman Catholic priests are pedophiles or teen hebephiles
(Sipes 1990).

Recently, I was consulted in a vast multioffender-multivictim
sexual abuse case in a rural area just outside of Ottawa. I examined
one of the first alleged perpetrators arrested in a case that to date
has led to 65 persons being charged for sexual abuse of more than
275 victims. I evaluated this mildly mentally retarded man who

initially denied any sexual involvement with children. However, once he had completed a sexual behaviors assessment and was found to be a pedophile, he admitted extensive sexual abuse. The assessment included physiological testing of sexual arousal, which clearly showed him to be pedophilic and coercive in his erotic preference for children of both sexes. He admitted to the ritualized sexual abuse of children and even infants younger than age 2 years. He described episodes where groups of men victimized children repeatedly, often with women in a spectator role. In this case, satanic rituals were suspected but no corroborating evidence was found. The investigation included exhumation to search for evidence of infant victims of satanic sacrifices (W. Cole and Bradford 1993).

The sexual abuse of children is a serious problem, and it extends far beyond what we realize, although this abuse is unlikely to include ritualized sexual abuse in the sense that it has origins in satanism. It is possible that a greater number of Christians are involved in sexual abuse of children than satanists. One only has to keep up-to-date with the media to note that the number of priests who have been convicted of repeated sexual abuse of children is greater than those with any connection to satanism.

"Expert Witnesses" Not Always Experts

In the court system, professionals, including myself (who assess sexual behaviors by using questionnaires, hormonal measures, and reliable and valid physiological measures of sexual arousal), have, for the most part, refrained from testifying in courts regarding someone's guilt or innocence by using these techniques. Yet, at the same time, investigations of sexual abuse of children and adults that are contaminated by a lack of any scientific method or validity and by therapeutic suggestion have been routinely allowed in the courtroom.

The qualifications of persons evaluating children for RA, and lack of standards defining how examinations should be conducted, is another serious problem. I believe that only child psychiatrists and Ph.D.-level psychologists should be allowed to examine children who report RA and should be required to have forensic training.

Another important issue is defining the word *ritualistic*, a term often associated with satanism. In more generic terms, ritualistic means a repeated act or series of acts. These acts can be sexual or other acts. To prevent confusion about ritualized sexual abuse, it is better defined as a multioffender-multivictim sexual abuse. This latter term will fare much better in the courts than will the term *satanic ritualistic abuse.*

The drastic influence of social mores on behavior and psychiatric attitudes has been described throughout the history of psychiatry. We should remember these stories, such as the witch trials in Salem, Massachusetts, in 1692. Young women in trancelike states exhibited bizarre behavior and somatic hallucinations, even while the witch trials were going on in the courtroom (Gardner 1991). Although there was no corroborating evidence of the accused being witches, those who denied complicity were executed. After the executions, some of the young women later admitted that their accusations were false. The accused who admitted complicity were spared execution. A number of authors have recently drawn analogies between the Salem witch trials and current child sexual abuse cases in the courtrooms of the United States and Canada (Gardner 1991).

Hypnosis and the Court System

It is critical that therapists understand the forensic aspects of hypnotically recalled and spontaneously recovered memories of previously dissociated traumas. The court system functions on credibility and uncovers facts; based on these facts, the court seeks to resolve disputes, including custody or criminal cases. Currently, hypnosis and suggestibility are being used to help witnesses or victims remember forgotten details of the trauma of sexual abuse (i.e., delayed recall). These witnesses subsequently testify not only to the abuse but also against the perpetrators who victimized them. Testimony of the witnesses often results from hypnotically induced recall or from suggestion in highly suggestible individuals for whom formal hypnosis is not used. The American Medical Association (AMA) Council on Scientific Affairs (1985) examined the scientific status of hypnotically refreshed recollection and reported on its use in the courtroom. I served as a resource person on this panel, which raised important questions about the credibility of suggestible patients who have been treated through hypnosis and other techniques inducing trance or hypnotic states. There is no doubt that hypnosis can be used as a therapeutic tool; in fact, the AMA has recognized hypnosis as a therapeutic modality since 1958. However, hypnosis, when used to refresh memory, is controversial.

Courts have taken opposing positions to testimony by witnesses who have undergone hypnosis. Some allow hypnotically refreshed memory to be included in an individual's testimony, whereas other courts have ruled that any individual who has ever been hypnotized is not allowed to testify on a matter addressed in hypnosis. The AMA Council on Scientific Affairs evaluated scientific evidence of the effect of hypnosis on memory, specifically heterohypnosis. In heterohypnosis, a hypnotist and a subject interact. Autohypnosis and self-induced hypnosis also can have significant effects on memory but were not specifically examined by the council.

The council reviewed clinical case studies, field reports, and pertinent literature reviews examining hypnosis and its effects on memory, including the following topics:

- Memory during hypnotic age regression
- Hypnotic enhancement of rote memory
- Hypnotic enhancement of recognition memory for meaningful and complex material
- Hypnotic enhancement of recall memory for meaningful and complex materials
- Hypnotic enhancement of memory for analog events

Organic Amnesia Versus Psychogenic Amnesia

It is important that therapists have a basic understanding of organic and functional amnesia and memory functioning. Organic amnesia generally refers to organic injury to the brain that interferes with an individual's ability to lay down a memory trace. Anterograde amnesia and retrograde amnesia are two types of organic amnesia. Functional amnesia, also known as psychogenic amnesia or dissociative amnesia (the term *psychogenic* is henceforth used), occurs without any evidence of underlying organic brain pathology and is mostly related to a traumatic event. Psychogenic amnesia is almost without exception a retrograde amnesia, that is, the inability to recall information that occurred before or around the precipitating event. Forensic psychiatrists are confronted, almost daily, with psychogenic amnesia of a retrograde type. Forensic psychiatrists have enormous experience in evaluating psychogenic amnesia. Traditionally, recovering psychogenic amnesia has been done through hypnosis, Sodium Amytal interviews, and, most commonly, repeated interviews and confrontation. There is a considerable body of forensic literature and nonforensic literature on recovering psychogenic amnesia. Another particularly important issue is malingered amnesia and how it can be differentiated from true amnesia. Against this background of organic and psychogenic amnesia, the AMA panel studied the role of hypnosis in refreshing memories.

Problems With Hypnosis

In a real-life situation, it is impossible to measure the accuracy of hypnotically recalled and spontaneously recovered memories, which makes research very difficult or impossible. In the majority of cases, it is impossible to be absolutely certain of what actually happened. Furthermore, it is the nature of the memory process that the more time passes between the incident and recovered memories of the incident, the more the accuracy of the memories deteriorates. In other words, there is no gold standard. Even in a situation of full consciousness without the contamination of hypnosis, the accuracy of recall as time passes is questionable. Therefore, it would seem logical that either suggested or hypnotic memory recall would be an even less clear and relevant account of what actually happened.

Hypnosis traditionally has been used to refresh memory in two ways: 1) age regression and 2) suggestion. With hypnotic age regression, patients are induced to behave in a manner appropriate to the age when the traumatic event occurred. Usually, the memories then are related to posttraumatic events. In sexual abuse investigations (most commonly child sexual abuse in adults), patients under hypnosis are urged to relive the highly emotional event. Freud, who first studied hypnotically recalled memories of childhood sexual abuse, initially was convinced that his patients recalled actual events. He subsequently concluded that the events did not actually occur, and although the emotional responses of his patients may have been real, they originated from a combination of fantasies, desires and fears, and actual memories (American Medical Association 1985).

Controlled studies have not supported the accuracy of hypnotically recalled memory during age regression, although scientific data are not conclusive. The hypnotic technique most commonly used to suggest increased recall has been the television technique (Reiser 1980). Through hypnosis, the therapist suggests to the subject that memory is organized like a video camera that can be switched on, and previous events can be observed and memories maintained indefinitely. This video camera thesis is completely inconsistent with research on memory and is no longer considered accurate.

Another controversial issue is that hypnosis can create false memories. When a patient is hypnotized, a therapist can easily suggest that certain events occurred. The patient then may respond by confabulation. Reviews of the scientific literature showed that there is no scientific evidence that hypnosis increases the recall of rote memory or that recognition memory is in any way enhanced (American Medical Association 1985). A review of the literature on hypnotically enhanced recall of complex material found that there was some evidence that hypnosis could increase the recall of a number of meaningful items. However, the problem was that hypnosis increased the overall production of material but not accuracy (American Medical Association 1985). In fact, it was found that patients simply confabulated to fill in anything that could not be remembered. Hypnosis appears to enhance the production of recall memory; however, confabulation plays a role, and there is no way to differentiate between a true memory and a false one.

A classic study by Stalnaker and Riddle (1932) showed that hypnosis could help subjects remember poetry learned many years ago. In this study, subjects remembered more about the poem when they were in a hypnotic state as opposed to a nonhypnotic state. Later in this study, it was found that participants simply filled in words in a plausible but inaccurate way. In other words, con-fabulation helped to produce recall of complex material, but recall was inaccurate (Stalnaker and Riddle 1932). Similar results were found in the literature on hypnosis and memory of analog events and real-life events. Again, it was found that hypnosis increased recall; however, there was an increase in both accurate and false memories, demonstrating the limitations of experimental research in this area.

The AMA panel also recognized, even in nonhypnotized sub-jects, that eyewitness testimony was extremely vulnerable to bias through leading questions and other techniques. Even more sig-nificant was the discovery that as soon as hypnosis was introduced, vulnerability to the effects of leading questions and bias was mag-nified and had a powerful influence on individuals. It was not clear whether the hypnotic trance itself or simply an individual's level of hypnotizability made him or her vulnerable to suggestion. Cur-rently, the latter is considered more likely to be true.

The panel concluded that it could not support the use of hyp-nosis to enhance memory of analog events because hypnosis can lead to false recollection and confabulation, particularly in both crime victims and witnesses who experience traumatic amnesia or posttraumatic stress disorder. This issue recently has been re-viewed in the book *Trance on Trial* (Scheflin and Shapiro 1989). The above mentioned AMA panel concluded that when hypnosis is used to enhance recall

- Hypnosis produces recollections that are not substantially differ-ent from nonhypnotically induced recollections.
- Hypnosis produces recollections that are more inaccurate than nonhypnotically induced recollections.
- Hypnosis frequently results in more information being recalled, but this information is both accurate and inaccurate. The sub-stantial increase of recalled information includes both true and false memories, and there is no way of knowing which is the accurate memory.

The scientific literature also showed that hypnosis caused inac-curate memories, but individuals confidently would report these false memories as accurate. Clearly, inaccurate memories are of the utmost danger when these individuals testify in court (Putnam 1979; Zelig and Beidleman 1981). A basic premise in law is that credibility is the responsibility of the fact finder, which is either the judge or the jury. In a courtroom, the credibility of a witness often is based on the fact finder's observation of the performance of the witness. The fact finder's observations are nonscientific, subjective perceptions of whether the witness is lying and of his or her emotional responses, body language, and other factors while he or she is testifying. An important factor is the degree of confidence that an individual portrays in recounting memories; it has an enormously powerful influence on the fact finder. If a witness has been hypnotized and is able to recount false memories with a high level of confidence, it is obvious that the entire court system could be corrupted.

Hypnosis, through the medium of suggestion, can produce memories of events that did not occur, and these memories can be triggered by subtle cues aside from leading questions (Loftus 1979). According to the AMA Council on Scientific Affairs (1985), "to the extent that a suspicion may be transformed into a vivid pseudo-memory in hypnosis, there may be serious consequences to the legal process where testimony is based on material that is elicited from a witness who has been hypnotized for the purpose of refreshing recollection about the incident in question" (p. 1922). The council, when studying amnesia in defendants and hypnosis used to overcome amnesia, determined that corroboration is very important because even individuals under the influence of hypnosis can knowingly lie. As a forensic psychiatrist, I have considerable experience in dealing with amnesia of defendants and throughout my career have used various techniques to counteract amnesia, including Sodium Amytal, hypnosis, and lie detection techniques such as polygraphs and voice stress analysis (Bradford and Smith 1980; Lynch and Bradford 1981). Although forensic psychiatrists have focused on differentiating organic and psychogenic amnesia, the general conclusion has been that in practice, differentiating these types of amnesia is very difficult if not impossible. In addition, the reliability or veracity of hypnotically induced memories cannot be scientifically verified with any degree of accuracy (Bradford 1994;

Bradford and Smith 1980; Lynch and Bradford 1980).

The American Society of Clinical Hypnosis Committee on Hypnosis and Memory (1995) published its opinions on forensic hypnosis. I strongly recommend that everyone in the forensic arena who is interested in repressed or recovered memories read these guidelines for clinicians.

Amnesia and the Polygraph

Detecting amnesia by psychophysiological measures (e.g., polygraph), in my experience, appeared to be useful in delineating alcohol or drug-induced amnesia, which would be considered genuine or real amnesia as opposed to feigned or dissociative amnesia. The charges brought against an individual did not affect the type of amnesia; that is, genuine or deceptive amnesia was spread evenly across various offenses. Polygraph determinations compared with length of alcohol and drug abuse history showed that genuine amnesia as reported by polygraphs correlated well with the length of the consumption of alcohol and drugs, indicating the greater probability of organic brain syndrome and the amnesia reported by the subject was truthful. The opposite is also true: when there is less abuse of drugs or alcohol, the chance of organic brain syndrome causing amnesia is less likely and the probability that memory is feigned is greater. Although this converse theory cannot be generalized, it becomes important when one considers that the victims of sexual abuse are principally females who are also less likely to use alcohol, and it follows that their amnesia is more likely to be dissociative in the majority of cases. The incidence of dissociative disorders, including multiple personality disorder, is common in females who have been sexually abused, which further supports this contention. If there are differences in suggestibility and vulnerability to dissociative disorder and multiple personality disorder in females compared with males, and there are no clear answers to this issue, then one must consider the impact of dissociative disorder in the victims of sexual abuse and its impact on amnesia and accurate recall of delayed memories. Therapists should not hold any preconceived biases; however, a number of influences clearly affect the accuracy of recall, even without hypnosis.

Using Hypnosis With Witnesses and Victims

The AMA Council on Scientific Affairs (1985) made the following five recommendations:

1. The use of hypnosis with witnesses and victims to enhance recall should be limited to the investigative process. Corroboration is of the utmost importance.
2. Before inducing hypnosis, a detailed history and evaluation of the patient should be done, and the individual's recollections should be obtained without leading questions. Material that cannot be remembered should not be accepted at face value but should be explored carefully to determine the degree or extent of the memory or the amnesia. Repeated interviewing with nonleading questions and without suggestion may assist in recall efforts and may result in accurate recall. Only after these repeated interviews should hypnosis be considered, and all precautions should be taken to avoid leading questions or suggestion.
3. Hypnosis should be conducted only by a psychiatrist or psychologist skilled in the clinical, investigative use of hypnosis who is aware of the legal implications in using hypnosis for investigative purposes within the jurisdiction in which he or she practices. In addition, a complete videotaped, precise written record should be kept. (These records may be relevant if sexual abuse victims are evaluated by poorly qualified, untrained individuals.)
4. Only the psychiatrist or psychologist and patient should be present during hypnosis because subtle cuing could occur from other persons in the room. (Cuing from others present excludes cuing that could come from the psychiatrist or psychologist, although such cuing might be recorded on the videotape.)
5. Whatever form of hypnosis is used, one episode of free narrative recall should be made first, and it should be made clear to the patient that saying "I don't know" is acceptable.

Other recommendations included that the medical responsibility for the hypnotized patient not be forsaken because an investigation is being conducted. Assessing the patient's response to terminating hypnosis and posthypnotic discussion of the session were also seen as critical. Further research on psychogenic amnesia and memory was recommended.

The council concluded that recollections obtained during hypnosis can involve confabulation and pseudomemories and not only fail to be more accurate, but also actually appear to be less reliable than nonhypnotic recall. The use of hypnosis with witnesses or victims may have serious consequences for the legal process, when testimony is based on material that is elicited from a witness who has been hypnotized for the purpose of refreshing recollection (American Medical Association 1985).

Although this conclusion is relatively narrow in terms of sexual abuse and ritualized sexual abuse, the same principles should apply to delayed recall of previously dissociated traumas.

Problems With Memory Accuracy

Delayed memory recall also is based largely on childhood memories. There is considerable concern about the accuracy of these memories even during childhood (i.e., not delayed) for various reasons. There is potential for error at all stages of the memory process: reception, registration, retention, and recall (Bradford and Smith 1980) or, in other terms, encoding, retention, or retrieval (Johnson and Howell 1993). Children and adults have potential sources of error in all of these phases (Johnson and Howell 1993). There has been considerable research to evaluate children's performance in all of these stages of memory.

There are differences in information processing in children compared with adults, particularly differences in information retained or encoded (Johnson and Howell 1993; Yarmey and Kent 1980). On an age-related continuum, there appears to be little selectivity in the information processing of children. Loftus and Davies (1984) found that children's retention was more splintered than adults'. Others have reported similar findings in children younger than age 7 years (Chi 1976; Chi and Ceci 1986; Saywitz 1987). The issue is complex, although there appear to be age-related issues of error, including suggestibility (Ceci et al. 1987; C. D. Cole and Loftus 1987). Various types of age-related memory difficulties lead to errors in registration, attention, and recall. There is uncertainty about the accuracy of what is actually recalled at the time the memory trace is laid in childhood; when delayed recall is assisted by hypnosis and suggestibility, the potential for error is enormous, including (not exclusively) the production of vivid pseudomemories. However, the production of pseudomemories does not totally invalidate hypnotically recalled information. Without corroboration, delayed memory recall either hypnotically induced or occurring spontaneously should be seriously scrutinized.

Conclusion

Sadistic abuses are a reality in our society as evidenced by numerous convictions of pedophiles and hebephiles. Some of the victims can dissociate these memories until sometime in the future when, whether through flashbacks or other events, the abuses may be recalled in the therapy setting. Because of erroneous therapeutic techniques, and even unconscious cuing techniques, many false elements can be introduced inadvertently into memory recall. I suggest that therapists be properly trained and qualified before considering themselves competent to appear in court as expert witnesses.

Therapists must understand the potential difficulties in assessing the recall of previously repressed or dissociated traumas. Finally, they should be very aware of the influence of hypnosis and related techniques on the therapist-patient interaction, and they must know the laws in their jurisdictions pertaining to the acceptability of hypnotically assisted memory recall in the courtroom.

References

Abel GG, Mittleman MS, Becker JV: Sexual offenders: results of assessment and recommendations for treatment, in Clinical Criminology: Current Concepts. Edited by Ben-Aron MH, Hucker SJ, Webster CD. Toronto, Ontario, M & M Graphics, 1985, pp 191–207

American Medical Association Council on Scientific Affairs: Council report: scientific status of refreshing recollection by the use of hypnosis. JAMA 253:1918–1923, 1985

American Society of Clinical Hypnosis Committee on Hypnosis and Memory: Clinical Hypnosis and Memory: Guidelines for Clinicians and for Forensic Hypnosis. Des Plaines, IL, American Society of Clinical Hypnosis, 1995

Bradford JMW: Amnesia and Amytal interviews, in Principles and Practice of Forensic Psychiatry. Edited by Rosner R. New York, Chapman & Hall, 1994, pp 494–496

Bradford JMW, Smith SM: Amnesia and homicide: the Padola case and a study of thirty cases. Bull Am Acad Psychiatry Law 8:219–231, 1980

Bradford JMW, Boulet J, Pawlak A: The paraphilias: a multiplicity of deviant behaviors. Can J Psychiatry 30:104–108, 1992

Ceci SJ, Ross DF, Toglia MP: Age differences in suggestibility: narrowing the uncertainty, in Children's Eyewitness Testimony. Edited by Ceci SJ, Toglia MP, Ross DF. New York, Springer-Verlag, 1987, pp 79–91

Chi MTH: Short-term memory limitations in children: capacity or processing deficits. Memory and Cognition 4:201–210, 1976

Chi MTH, Ceci SJ: Content, knowledge and reorganization of memory. Child Development and Behavior 20:1–37, 1986

Cole CD, Loftus E: The memory of children, in Children's Eyewitness Testimony. Edited by Ceci SJ, Toglia MP, Ross DF. New York, Springer-Verlag, 1987

Cole W, Bradford J: Multi-offender, multi-victim sexual abuse assessments. Paper presented at the meeting of the American Academy of Psychiatry and the Law, San Antonio, TX, October 1993

Committee on Sexual Offences Against Children and Youths: Report of the Committee on Sexual Offences Against Children and Youths, Vols 1 and 2 (J 2-50/1984E). Ottawa, Canada, Canadian Government Publishing Centre, 1984

Franklin E, Wright W: Sins of the Father. New York, Ballantine Books, 1993

Gardner RA: Sex Abuse Hysteria: Salem Witch Trials Revisited. Longwood, NJ, Creative Therapeutics Press, 1991

Johnson EK, Howell RJ: Memory processes in children: implications for investigations of alleged child sexual abuse. Bull Am Acad Psychiatry Law 21:213–226, 1993

Lanning KV: Satanic, or cults, ritualistic crime: a law enforcement perspective. Royal Canadian Mounted Police Gazette 3:615, 1991

Lanning KV: Investigators Guide to Allegations of "Ritual" Child Abuse. Washington, DC, U.S. Federal Bureau of Investigation, 1992

Loftus EF: Eyewitness Testimony. Cambridge, MA, Harvard University Press, 1979

Loftus EF, Davies GM: Distortion. Journal of Social Issues 4:51–67, 1984

Lynch B, Bradford JMW: Amnesia: its detection by psychophysiological measures. Bull Am Academy Psychiatry Law 8:288–297, 1980

Putnam WH: Hypnosis and distortions in eyewitness memory. Int J Clin Exp Hypn 27:437–448, 1979

Reiser M: Handbook of Investigative Hypnosis. Los Angeles, CA, Lehi Publishing, 1980

Saywitz KJ: Children's testimony: age-related patterns of memory errors, in Children's Eyewitness Testimony. Edited by Ceci SJ, Toglia MP, Ross DF. New York, Springer-Verlag, 1987, pp 36–52

Scheflin AW, Shapiro JL: Trance on Trial. New York, Guilford, 1989

Sipes R: A Secret World: Sexuality in the Search for Celibacy. New York, Brunner/Mazel, 1990

Stalnaker JM, Riddle EE: The effect of hypnosis on long delayed recall. J Gen Psychol 6:429–440, 1932

Timnick L: 22% in a survey were child abuse victims. Los Angeles Times, August 25, 1985, p 1

Yarmey AD, Kent J: Eyewitness identification by elderly and young adults. Law and Human Behavior 4:359–371, 1980

Zelig M, Beidleman WB: The investigative use of hypnosis: a word of caution. Int J Clin Exp Hypn 29:401–412, 1981

CHAPTER 11

Teen Involvement in the Occult

Robert J. Simandl

About 10 years ago, I was asked to develop a program to educate law enforcement personnel on the topic of ritual abuse. My own background in this area began at a training session for gang investigations in Los Angeles, California. For several years after this training session, I had attended lectures on my own time. Books on the subject of ritual abuse were not available, and it was difficult locating resources pertaining to this subject. Even today, there are limited books on ritual abuse, especially on the issue of teenage involvement. After almost a decade in this field, I encounter new information daily.

The field of ritual abuse can be divided into four different levels or categories. These categories are flexible and could be expanded as we encounter more information. The four levels are

1. Experimental teen dabbler group
2. Self-styled or nontraditional group
3. Organized traditional group
4. Occultic networking group

The first category, experimental teen dabblers, refers to adolescents who exhibit ritual behaviors but do not have family involvement. In the second category, self-styled individuals or groups engage in ritualistic activity as an outcome of their own bizarre behavior and are not associated with any other group. The third organized traditional group includes networking as an integral component. Included here are the reported intergenerational and nonfamily participation groups who use rituals to abuse children and commit other illegal acts (as may other categories). The final group, the occultic networking group, is said to use ritual activity to control others for the purpose of obtaining power and money through illegal modes. It is supposedly more widespread than the other three groups.

The purpose of this chapter is to focus on teenagers who dabble with the symbols and rituals associated with satanism and other areas of the occult, or the experimental teen dabbler group. Although the problems with this group are not as prominent as street gang problems in the United States, the growing phenomenon of teenage dabblers is a major concern (Wheeler and Wood 1988) and a problem for both urban and rural populations.

The term *dabbler* may be misleading, as I have discovered in my work that these teens are killing themselves, their parents, and others. I may eventually change my terminology because my conclusion is that the behavior of this group is often more serious than just dabbling.

Dabbler/Experimentalist Behavior Indicators

Based on investigations of teen dabblers, I compiled in 1994 the following list of common behaviors noted in those involved in ritual practices. The list was formulated for investigators and therapists to indicate warning signs possibly requiring intervention. If an individual displays these warning signs, it does not necessarily prove he or she is active in ritual activity; it may imply that he or she is vulnerable or susceptible and that intervention could be warranted. Intervention at early stages may revert the process of ritual involvement.

1. Suicide/attempted suicide
2. Undue fascination with death, torture, and suicide
3. Violent and aggressive behavior directed toward parents, siblings, and authority figures
4. Obnoxious antisocial behavior
5. Alienation from family and religion

6. Self-mutilation and tattooing
7. Fascination for edged weapons
8. Bizarre cruelty
9. Drug and alcohol abuse
10. Drastic change in grades
11. High truancy rate
12. Leaving home at unusual hours
13. New peer group
14. Compulsive interest in occult material, fantasy role games, and films and videos (all with themes of death, torture, and suicide)

If a number of these warning signs are observed, do not confront the individual; do not confiscate any materials, unless they are contraband; and do contact a knowledgeable person or team to evaluate the individual.

Crime Scene and Homicide Investigations

Crime scene and homicide investigations have uncovered the following scenarios and materials suggesting satanic ritualized activity has taken place (Kahaner 1988; Pulling 1989):

- Mockery of Christian symbols (inverted cross, vandalized Christian articles)
- Silver instruments (amulets, knives, chalices)
- Candles or drippings
- Unusual drawings or symbols on walls or floors (hexagram, pentagram, horn of death)
- Nondiscernible alphabet (sometimes a so-called witch's alphabet)
- Animal mutilations, including specific body parts such as anus, heart, tongue, ears, front teeth, front legs (hoofs), and genitals
- Animal parts and bones forming signs and symbols
- Absence of blood in the sacrificed animal
- Stone or metal altar containing artifacts such as black candles, white-handled knife, salt, and knotted colored cords
- Clay figures, effigies, and voodoo dolls stuck with pins or otherwise mutilated
- Bowls of powder or colored salts, drugs, or herbs

- Skulls with or without candles
- Bones (possibly taken from graves) such as femur, tibia, index finger, skull, and others
- Hooded robes (sometime sweatshirts), especially black, white, and scarlet
- Jewelry such as amulets
- Colored plastic drop cloths
- Rooms draped in red or black
- Books on satanism, such as *Majick in Theory and Practice* (Crowley 1976) and the *Satanic Bible* (LaVey 1969), or a diary of ritual activities, also called a "book of shadows"; videotapes, record albums, or cassettes with satanic references
- Bells or gongs
- Oils or incense found on a cadaver suspected to have been used in a ritual ceremony
- Body painted or tied up
- Neck wounds (likely to have rendered the victim unconscious)
- Branding-iron marks or burn marks
- Ritualistic symbols carved on body
- Candle wax drippings found on a body used in a ritual
- Human or animal feces consumed, smeared on body, or found in body cavities such as mouth, eyes, and nose
- Stomach contents of urine, drugs, wine, potions, and blood
- Evidence of bloodletting
- Semen in, on, or near body cavities
- Lungs filled with blood, smoke, or liquid
- Scarring between index finger and thumb or inside wrist
- Missing body parts such as heart, genitals, left or right hand, tongue, and index finger
- Stab wounds
- Masks or costumes
- Crystals
- Posters of mythological beings or heavy-metal rock groups
- Martial arts weaponry, paraphernalia, or clothing

Discovery of these items or reference to these scenarios in an adolescent's dialogue, writings, or drawings may indicate some degree of ritual involvement.

Reported Criminal Activities Committed by Ritual Groups

In addition to ritual activities, other criminal activities have been consistently discovered and reported to be committed by all four categories of ritual groups. The following is a list of crimes most frequently committed by ritual groups:

- Murder
- Child abuse
- Sexual assault
- Physical assault
- Pornography
- Child prostitution
- Drug distribution and sales
- Arson for destruction
- Arson for profit
- Fraud
- Kidnapping of derelicts, runaways, homeless, and illegal immigrants
- Money laundering
- Gunrunning
- Burglary
- Illegal and forced abortions

Again, references to or evidence of the above activities in combination with the previously mentioned behavioral indicators may be, but are not always, signs that an adolescent is involved in ritual activity.

Case Examples

Although there is no stereotypical teen experimentalist, there are some common characteristics. Typically, the ages range from 10 to 20 years; both sexes are involved. Some of the youths are intelligent, some are underachievers, and most come from middle- and upper-class families, although not exclusively.

The following case example illustrates teenage involvement in a ritual group in a Hispanic community in Chicago. The teenager's ritualistic behavior resulted in his suicide at age 19 years.

Case 1

Jose had been a straight A student. During an investigation of his home, materials were found suggesting ritual involvement. There were indications that he had an obsession with death, torture, and suicide. In response to a class assignment to write of one's plans for the future, this young man wrote about his impending suicide plans. The school newspaper found it worthy enough to publish, but unfortunately no one found it worthy enough to consider seriously as a possible cry for help. His drawings, writings, and actions dealing with mutilations and suicide were considered merely a creative fad. These indicators did not suddenly develop overnight; rather, there were warning signs that should have been deciphered long before the suicide.

Jose's suicide is a prime example of the potential danger of ignoring and denying warning signs. Considering warning signs as just a fad can be a fatal mistake. All too often the philosophy of teens who become obsessed with rituals with satanic overtones is one of violence, self-destruction, and eventual suicide.

This case might have ended there except for a strange coincidence that happened later that same year. I was first alerted to another case by an article in a Chicago newspaper.

Case 2

Juan, a 17-year-old Hispanic, had stabbed his sister 48 times, then poured bleach on her. He also had forced her to drink ammonia. Finally, he sprayed her with a bug pesticide. This vicious attack was the result of a disagreement that they had. My immediate reaction was that there was likely more to this story than a simple family argument. Because I was a youth officer in Chicago, it was not too surprising that this young man ended up in my station. The violent-crime detective who arrested him conferred with me about his findings in this case. Much of the information had a ring of familiarity. I then discovered that Juan was the brother of Jose, in Case 1, who had committed suicide earlier in the year.

Like his brother, Juan had been involved in ritual behaviors, which he delved into even deeper after the suicide of Jose. No follow-up counseling had been done with this family to identify indicators of ritual behavior. The warning signs were clearly there, but even with the suicide of his brother, these signs were denied and ignored. I asked Juan if he somehow got power from his brother's suicide. His eyes rolled up, and with a gleam in them he answered, "Yeah!"

Certainly, there were indicators that this young man was urgently in need of intense therapy (Wheeler and Wood 1988). Problem behaviors that are ignored and allowed to get out of control can and do result in tragedies.

An attraction to ritual activity is not the sole problem for these youths. They also have been noted to have low self-esteem, a morbid curiosity beyond the norm, boredom, and difficulty relating to peers (Wheeler and Wood 1988). Therapy is crucial for these teenagers. In my opinion, rebellion is the driving force in teenage involvement in ritual activities. Each generation has its unique form of rebellion. In most cases, the infatuation with ritualistic symbols and activities is just a fad and can be overlooked; in a smaller number of teens, this behavior may get out of control quickly and must be addressed. Precipitating factors that may act as catalysts to teen ritual involvement include the death of a loved one, an overzealous religious family, and lack of peer acceptance.

There is a specific pattern of development when a teenager becomes more deeply involved in ritual activity. The end result often is death, generally by suicide. The developmental sequence is based on actual cases that have occurred in the United States: First, the interest in rituals is piqued, then progresses to group involvement. The teens start collecting satanic literature. Soon, the performance of rituals begins; these rituals include cutting themselves and drinking the blood. Getting tattoos is not uncommon. Next, the sacrifice of small animals may take place. For some, this leads to the sacrifice of even larger animals. Some groups become bored with animal sacrifice and may discuss the ultimate sacrifice: human beings.

The following case demonstrates this developmental sequence.

It occurred a number of years ago in a small town in the midwestern United States.

Case 3

Four teenagers were becoming more deeply involved in ritual activity. Their behaviors were tolerated because of the hope and expectation that this activity was a fad that would soon end. As the sequence progressed, they became bored with animal sacrifices, and they felt they would like to experience a human sacrifice. They decided to sacrifice one of their own group. In October, they devised a death contract, which they signed with their own blood. In December, a member to be sacrificed had been selected. The procedure began with the ceremonial sacrifice of a cat. All four of the participants drank a mixture of wine and blood and urine from the cat. The group proceeded by bludgeoning the targeted young man with a baseball bat. They disposed of his body by throwing it in a well along with the body of the cat for symbolic purposes. This human sacrifice had been the culmination of a 2-year sequential progression of this group's ritual activities. It left one 19-year-old dead and three 16-year-olds charged with murder. The contract signed in blood discounted one of the teen's attempts to plead insanity. They were all convicted and parole was denied. The unspoken tragedy in this case was that there could have been therapeutic intervention, given the warning signs apparent to any informed professional.

In conceptualizing the group members in this case, one might suppose that the teenagers wore heavy-metal rock group shirts and dressed in black with inverted crosses dangling from their ears. This supposition could not be farther from the truth. In fact, the leader was the senior class president in that small midwestern town. One must go beyond appearances and focus on behavioral indicators and problems. More often than not, teens dressed in heavy-metal garb are simply emulating one of their favorite rock groups and are not at all involved in ritual activities.

The belief of teens dabbling in these occult rituals is that if they kill themselves, they will return as stronger beings. Because of this belief, the risk of suicide must be a major focus of concern in therapy. This reincarnation philosophy helps explain the undue fascination with death, torture, weaponry, and suicide. At times, the purpose of self-mutilation is merely to endure pain and to obtain blood from their own arms or legs to use in ceremonies. Symbols such as 666, the "sign of the beast" (occasionally represented as FFF, the sixth letter of the alphabet), and inverted crucifixes are important in some ceremonies. Teens at times may tattoo these symbols on their bodies (Wheeler and Wood 1988). Not all teenagers who draw occult or satanic symbols in their notebooks are involved in ritual activities. All factors should be reviewed objectively before suspecting the possibility of ritual involvement.

What if a teenager does exhibit the behavioral indicators of ritual activity? The initial procedure is to answer four basic questions to ascertain the level of involvement:

1. How did this behavior start?
2. Who is involved?
3. Is there a group involvement?
4. Is there a leader?

It is important to establish if the teenager became involved alone, with a number of like-minded teenagers, or with a family group. Other key elements to consider are whether the teen was lured into the ritual involvement and whether adults were involved in the process. A positive answer to the latter could move the teen's level of involvement out of an experimentalist group and into one of the other three groups mentioned earlier in this chapter. These four questions are sometimes not easily answered but are important in therapeutic strategies.

If a teenager conveys that he or she was introduced to ritual activity by attending a party, it is imperative to discover exactly what transpired at the party. If he or she describes situations that include free sex and drugs, suspicions should abound. Who offered free sex and drugs? The motives for these actions need to be contemplated. The therapist should determine whether these "generous" individuals were attempting to obtain an instant clientele in the drug market or to gain control for other purposes.

Patterns have been established for enticing teens into ritual activity. Often, teens refer to some area of woods or a house deemed

off-limits until they become better acquainted with other more established members. With time, they become accepted by these
members. Then the trap is sprung, and the new member is photo-
graphed or videotaped in a compromising situation either sexually
or under the influence of alcohol and/or drugs. Once the group
possesses a photograph or video of the person, the recruiters can
now control the person through blackmail. They use this new
member for criminal activity. Females often are used for sexual
activity. The criminal activities are not exclusively ritualistic. For
example, a group of 70 teens in the southern suburban area of Chicago includes youths from eight different towns. Their mutual
bond was the ritual practices, but their escapades included burglar-
izing gas stations and homes and drug trafficking.

Initiation is another phase in the recruitment pattern. There are
various types of initiations. A common initiation is to sacrifice a
family cat and then drink a mixture of the cat's blood, urine, and
wine. Without any therapeutic intervention, the acts progressively
worsen. The common element in all recruitment phases is a compulsive interest and obsession with the beliefs and rituals of the
group.

When a teenager is involved in ritual activity, there is a need
for an evaluation. The evaluation is based on the behavioral indicators, as well as materials in the individual's possession. Collecting
personal belongings such as occult materials and books is essential,
followed by a team effort to review these materials objectively. The
greater the obsession with rituals, the more serious the problem.
The evaluation will determine the level of involvement (beginning
stages or heavily involved).

Fantasy role-playing games are commonly found among the
personal effects of a teen involved in ritual activity; however, in my
opinion, the majority of youths who engage in these games are not
going to become involved in ritual activity. However, if they have
preexisting emotional problems and become obsessed with these
games, therapeutic intervention is warranted.

The same guidelines apply to music. Most youths who listen to
heavy-metal music will not become involved in ritual activity.
There is no debating the issue that the names of some groups, titles
of songs, album covers, and lyrics are inundated with ritual sym-

bolism that could sway vulnerable people, but the majority of teens today are not influenced by this symbolism (Raschke 1990).

Diaries found in the belongings of ritually active teens are an excellent source of vital information needed for an evaluation. Diaries also supply valuable information concerning death and suicide contracts, which hopefully are discovered ahead of the intended dates. Many contain a listing of other members. The nicknames listed are critical in identifying perpetrators and victims. Descriptions of rituals also have been discovered in diaries (also called a "book of shadows"). Various codes may be used in the diaries. It is important to be familiar with the unusual alphabets and writings commonly used in the diaries. Some commonly used alphabets are the runic alphabet, codes from *The Book of Runes* (Blum 1982), the Theban alphabet, and the witch's alphabet.

These books of shadows may be found in various forms. In some cases, it is a black-covered book with blank pages, which can be purchased in occult book stores. However, in my experience, the majority are simply spiral notebooks or composition books. More recently, home computers are being used to store diary entries. Often, diaries may give clues to the level of involvement. The most important place to examine for ritual paraphernalia is a youth's bedroom. When questioned about the contents of an adolescent's room, parents frequently respond, "I'm not allowed in his or her bedroom." I wish that I could introduce the parents who say this to other parents who regret staying out of their child's room—their son or daughter is now dead.

In addition to many fantasy role-playing games, ritually active teens possess certain computer programs or games. One program supplies a step-by-step guide on how to murder five or six people at a time. The program includes a list of various poisons and all of their ingredients, which are readily available. Not all teens who play these types of games are going to follow through on the instructions; however, important warning signs of ritual activity via computer should not be ignored. For example, a young man killed himself after writing a suicide note on his home computer. If his parents had been alert to such signs of ritual activity and intervened, perhaps they could have taken their son to therapy rather than to a morgue.

Another family, wealthy but dysfunctional, was unaware of the warning signs that their teenage daughter was ritually active. Her father admitted that she was participating in some "strange stuff" and had some "weird" friends. They would spend hours chanting in her bedroom. The family allowed it because they thought it was "just a phase." One morning, her father, investigating some unusually loud chanting from his daughter's bedroom at 2 A.M., was met with thrusts from a butcher knife by the hands of his daughter. He finally was convinced there was a problem that needed professional attention.

This particular girl had been an absolute genius and an artist. The unusual change in her drawings definitely sent up red flags. She demonstrated many of the behavioral indicators that were cause for concern and intervention. She had taught herself to read and write backward. She created her own fantasy role-playing games and possessed a satanic crossword puzzle. She also wrote from *The Book of Runes* (Blum 1982). At age 14, she had attempted suicide and was hospitalized in an adolescent unit. The hospital was prepared to handle behavioral, substance and alcohol abuse, and suicidal problems. However, the hospital staff was in complete denial about the ritual activity. The staff did not believe it occurred and preferred not to address this issue. After months of hospitalization, they released her with no improvement in her condition from the day that she was admitted to the unit. Obsessive and compulsive interests in death, torture, and suicide permeated this young lady's actions until her father finally got the point when she attacked him with a butcher knife, and he realized she needed help in overcoming her fascination with ritualism.

This family's case in many aspects demonstrates the urgent need for therapists to seek expert opinions when efforts have been exhaustive and have resulted in little success for a patient's recovery. Cases involving ritual activity may be quite complicated, and there is no reason for therapists to feel embarrassed by requesting assistance from other professionals. Using *The Book of Runes*, the girl wrote a secret message indicating that she again was planning to commit suicide on the next full moon. Secret messages need to be found, deciphered, and understood so that therapists can intervene before a ritually active teen commits suicide.

When patients involved in ritual activity are admitted to an inpatient psychiatric unit, professionals not trained in this area inadvertently could cause problems by displaying these patients' drawings or by including such patients in group discussions that could adversely influence other vulnerable patients. Without the proper training, therapists do not realize the influence that ritually active patients have on non-ritually involved patients.

Family Tree Information File

It is important for therapists to establish whether the teenager is in the experimentalist category or in one of the other three categories. If the teenager is in the nontraditional group, organized traditional group, or occultic networking group, one multipurpose tool that has proven to be quite useful when gathering information and organizing data is the family tree information file. A survivor of ritual abuse, in conjunction with a therapist, fills out the family tree. The information required for this form is vital statistics of family members, from grandparents through recent births, as well as close family friends. There is a section for documenting previous addresses and a section referring to medical health care providers, including hospitals and specialists.

The family tree program assists therapists and patients in organizing factual information and memories. Therapists are cautioned to monitor their patients' reactions when obtaining the information. The process often triggers memory recall and the emotions associated with them, which can be very distressful. Empathy and support are imperative. Survivors or patients are encouraged to answer as many questions as possible, but they are not expected to answer every question; they also should not contact other family members or close friends to answer the questions. Survivors often reveal an enormous quantity of factual information. The family tree enables the therapist to identify quickly to whom the survivor is referring when naming a particular person and the role that person has in the abusive situation.

Law enforcement agents like myself are limited in our capabilities to pursue criminal activities and abuses that were committed 25–30 years ago. However, as I perceive the situation, these abusers do not quit; they do not retire from this activity. Because abusers continue to abuse, the family tree program can assist therapists as well as law enforcement agencies. Studying the family tree may lead us to recognize children who are being abused. This early phase of abuse is when intervention from therapists and law enforcement agents is possible. Intervention with children who are being abused is the most productive route in preventing and curtailing further abuse and other criminal activities. If therapists and law enforcement agents do not intervene early, these children can be abandoned in psychiatric units, can die, or can become perpetrators of abuse themselves rather than survivors of abuse.

Although I have primarily discussed teenagers, I end this chapter with some new and pertinent changes to the law in Illinois on the ritual abuse of children. A major obstacle for law enforcement agents in our attempts to curtail ritual abuse of children is the law. In some states, laws are nonexistent, making intervention by professionals impossible. Louisiana, Missouri, Texas, Idaho (House Bill 817 of 1990), and Illinois (House Bill 3633 of 1992) have recognized this obstacle and passed legislation addressing ritual abuse of children. The Illinois Ritual Child Abuse Law (Public Law 87-67), effective in January 1993, is one of the most stringent laws in the United States.

In the 1980s, various professionals, including members of the Illinois House of Representatives and Senate, law enforcement personnel, and child protection, medical, and mental health personnel, encountered ritual child abuse cases in Illinois and discovered that preexisting laws were insufficient to protect children from horrendous acts. In efforts to alleviate this dilemma, legislation was enacted and amended. Preexisting laws for ritual mutilation and inducement to commit suicide obtained more stringent penalties when committed in ceremonial rites. In 1991, the Senate of the Eighty-Seventh General Assembly of Illinois adopted Senate Joint Resolution 20 (Rock/Grandberg). This resolution created a task force composed of 12 members (3 each appointed by the Senate President, Senate Majority Leader, Speaker of the House, and House Minority Leader) to study the issue of ritual child abuse in the state of Illinois and recommend legislation to the General Assembly. Public hearings were held in the capital, Springfield, and in Chicago in 1992 as a result of the resolution. Through research, the task force determined that ritual abuse crimes against children were indeed an issue to be addressed in Illinois. A comprehensive ritual child abuse bill was devised. The Ritual Child Abuse Bill passed through the Illinois House of Representatives and Senate and was signed into law by the governor, effective January 1, 1993 (Public Law 87-67).

There are several important elements of Public Law 87-67. The penalty for ritualized abuse of a child is a class I felony for the first offense. The second or subsequent conviction for ritualized abuse of a child is a class X felony for which the offender may be sentenced to a term of life imprisonment.

According to the law, a person is guilty of ritualized abuse of a child (anyone younger than age 18 years) when he or she commits any of the following acts with, upon, or in the presence of a child as part of a ceremony, rite, or any similar observance:

- Actually, or in simulation, tortures, mutilates, or sacrifices any warm-blooded animal or human being
- Forces ingestion, injection, or other application of any narcotic, drug, hallucinogen, or anesthetic for the purpose of dulling sensitivity, cognition, and recollection of, or resistance to, any criminal activity
- Forces ingestion, or external application, of human or animal urine, feces, flesh, blood, bones, body secretions, nonprescribed drugs, or chemical compounds
- Involves the child in a mock, unauthorized, or unlawful marriage ceremony with another person or representation of any force or deity, followed by sexual contact with the child
- Places a living child into a coffin or open grave containing a human corpse or remains
- Threatens death or serious harm to a child and his or her parents, family, pets, or friends, instilling a well-founded fear in the child that the threat will be carried out
- Unlawfully dissects, mutilates, or incinerates a human corpse

It is hoped that, as a consequence of the established laws, task forces will be created (including law enforcement investigators at various levels, prosecutors, and mental health, medical, and child protection professionals with the proper education) to review, investigate, and intervene objectively in these cases and ultimately curtail ritual abuse whether the victims are teenagers, children, or adults.

Conclusion

The purpose of this chapter is to alert therapists about ritualized abuse. Teen dabbling at times can lead to serious consequences; early intervention by therapists and law enforcement agents can prevent or curtail involvement in ritual activities. Therapists should not overreact to every teenager who displays an interest in events and activities that have satanic themes. Conversely, therapists must recognize the behavioral indicators for patients whose curiosity could be progressing to dangerous and even lethal experimentation with self-styled or mimicked satanic rituals. Finally, recent laws passed in Illinois help clarify ritual abuse as a crime.

References

Blum R: The Book of Runes. New York, St. Martin's Press, 1982

Crowley A: Majick in Theory and Practice. New York, Dover Publications, 1976

Kahaner L: Cults That Kill: Probing the Underworld of Occultic Crime. New York, Warner Books, 1988

LaVey AS: Satanic Bible. New York, Avon Books, 1969

Pulling P: The Devils Web: Who Is Stalking Your Children for Satan? Lafayette, LA, Huntington House, 1989

Raschke CA: Painted Black. San Francisco, CA, Harper & Row, 1990

Wheeler BR, Wood R: Assessments and interventions with adolescents involved in Satanism. Journal of Social Work 3:547–550, 1988

Statement on Memories of Sexual Abuse

American Psychiatric Association Board of Trustees

*T*his *Statement* is in response to the growing concern regarding memories of sexual abuse. The rise in reports of documented cases of child sexual abuse has been accompanied by a rise in reports of sexual abuse that cannot be documented. Members of the public, as well as members of mental health and other professions, have debated the validity of some memories of sexual abuse, as well as some of the therapeutic techniques which have been used. The American Psychiatric Association has been concerned that the passionate debates about these issues have obscured the recognition of a body of scientific evidence that underlies widespread agreement among psychiatrists regarding psychiatric treatment in this area. We are especially concerned that the public confusion and dismay over this issue and the possibility of false accusations not discredit the reports of patients who have indeed been traumatized by actual previous abuse. While much more needs to be known, this *Statement* summarizes information about this topic that is important for psychiatrists in their work with patients for whom sexual abuse is an issue.

Sexual abuse of children and adolescents leads to severe negative consequences. Child sexual abuse is a risk factor for many classes of psychiatric disorders, including anxiety disorders, affective disorders, dissociative disorders, and personality disorders.

Children and adolescents may be abused by family members, including parents and siblings, and by individuals outside of their families, including adults in trusted positions, (e.g., teachers, clergy, camp counsellors). Abusers come from all walks of life. There is no uniform "profile" or other method to accurately distinguish those who have sexually abused children from those who have not.

Children and adolescents who have been abused cope with the trauma by using a variety of psychological mechanisms. In some instances, these coping mechanisms result in a lack of conscious awareness of the abuse for varying periods of time. Conscious thoughts and feelings stemming from the abuse may emerge at a later date.

It is not known how to distinguish, with complete accuracy, memories based on true events from those derived from other sources. The following observations have been made:

- Human memory is a complex process about which there is a substantial base of scientific knowledge. Memory can be divided into four stages: input (encoding), storage, retrieval, and recounting. All of these processes can be influenced by a variety of factors, including developmental stage, expectations and knowledge base prior to an event; stress and bodily sensations experienced during an event; post-event questioning; and the experience and context of the recounting of the event. In addition, the retrieval and recounting of a memory can modify the form of the memory, which may influence the content and the conviction about the veracity of the memory in the future. Scientific knowledge is not yet precise enough to predict how a certain experience or factor will influence a memory in a given person.

- Implicit and explicit memory are two different forms of memory that have been identified. *Explicit memory* (also termed declarative memory) refers to the ability to consciously recall facts or events. *Implicit memory* (also termed procedural memory) refers to behavioral knowledge of an experience without conscious recall. A child who demonstrates knowledge of a skill (e.g., bicycle riding) without recalling how he/she learned it, or an adult who has an affective reaction to an event without understanding the basis for that reaction (e.g., a combat veteran who panics when he hears the sound of a helicopter, but cannot remember that he was in a helicopter crash which killed his best friend) are demonstrating implicit memories in the absence of explicit recall. This distinction between explicit and implicit memory is fundamental because they have been shown to be supported by different brain systems, and because their differentiation and identification may have important clinical implications.

- Some individuals who have experienced documented traumatic events may nevertheless include some false or inconsistent elements in their reports. In addition, hesitancy in making a report, and recanting following the report can occur in victims of documented abuse. Therefore, these seemingly contradictory findings do not exclude the possibility that the report is based on a true event.
- Memories can be significantly influenced by questioning, especially in young children. Memories also can be significantly influenced by a trusted person (e.g., therapist, parent involved in a custody dispute) who suggests abuse as an explanation for symptoms/problems, despite initial lack of memory of such abuse. It has also been shown that repeated questioning may lead individuals to report "memories" of events that never occurred.

It is not known what proportion of adults who report memories of sexual abuse were actually abused. Many individuals who recover memories of abuse have been able to find corroborating information about their memories. However, no such information can be found, or is possible to obtain, in some situations. While aspects of the alleged abuse situation, as well as the context in which the memories emerge, can contribute to the assessment, there is no completely accurate way of determining the validity of reports in the absence of corroborating information.

Psychiatrists are often consulted in situations in which memories of sexual abuse are critical issues. Psychiatrists may be involved in a variety of capacities, including as the treating clinician for the alleged victim, for the alleged abuser, or for other family member(s); as a school consultant; or in a forensic capacity.

Basic clinical and ethical principles should guide the psychiatrist's work in this difficult area. These include the need for role clarity. It is essential that the psychiatrist and the other involved parties understand and agree on the psychiatrist's role.

Psychiatrists should maintain an empathic, non-judgmental, neutral stance towards reported memories of sexual abuse. As in the treatment of all patients, care must be taken to avoid prejudging the cause of the patient's difficulties, or the veracity of the patient's reports. A strong prior belief by the psychiatrist that sexual abuse, or other factors, are or are not the cause of the patient's problems is likely to interfere with appropriate assessment and treatment. Many individuals who have experienced sexual abuse have a history of not being believed by their parents, or others in whom they have put their trust. Expression of disbelief is likely to cause the patient further pain and decrease his/her willingness to seek needed psychiatric treatment. Similarly, clinicians should not exert pressure on patients to believe in events that may not have occurred, or to prematurely disrupt important relationships or make other important decisions based on these speculations. Clinicians who have not had the training necessary to evaluate and treat patients with a broad range of psychiatric disorders are at risk of causing harm by providing inadequate care for the patient's psychiatric problems and by increasing the patient's resistance to obtaining and responding to appropriate treatment in the future. In addition, special knowledge and experience are necessary to properly evaluate and/or treat patients who report the emergence of memories during the use of specialized interview techniques (e.g., the use of hypnosis or Amytal), or during the course of litigation.

The treatment plan should be based on a complete psychiatric assessment, and should address the full range of the patient's clinical needs. In addition to specific treatments for any primary psychiatric condition, the patient may need help recognizing and integrating data that informs and defines the issues related to the memories of abuse. As in the treatment of patients with any psychiatric disorder, it may be important to caution the patient against making major life decisions during the acute phase of treatment. During the acute and later phases of treatment, the issues of breaking off relationships with important attachment figures, of pursuing legal actions, and of making public disclosures may need to be addressed. The psychiatrist should help the patient assess the likely impact (including emotional) of such decisions, given the patient's overall clinical and social situation. Some patients will be left with unclear memories of abuse and no corroborating information. Psychiatric treatment may help these patients adapt to the uncertainty regarding such emotionally important issues.

The intensity of public interest and debate about these topics should not influence psychiatrists to abandon their commitment to basic principles of ethical practice, delineated in *The Principles of Medical Ethics With Annotations Especially Applicable to Psychiatry*. The following concerns are of particular relevance:

- Psychiatrists should refrain from making public statements about the veracity or other features of individual reports of sexual abuse.
- Psychiatrists should vigilantly assess the impact of their conduct on the boundaries of the doctor/patient relationship. This is especially critical when treating patients who are seeking care for conditions that are associated with boundary violations in their past.

The APA will continue to monitor developments in this area in an effort to help psychiatrists provide the best possible care for their patients.

This statement was approved by the Board of Trustees of the American Psychiatric Association on December 12, 1993.

Index

*Page numbers printed in **boldface** type refer to tables or figures.*